AF765593

ME, MY SON AND MUSCULAR DYSTROPHY

How I Improved
My Son's Health and Muscle Strength
with Three Simple and Natural Methods

Clémentine Ynna

DISCLAIMER

The author of this document believes that a natural and holistic approach to health and maintaining balance in the human body are of utmost importance to experience energy, vitality and dynamic health throughout life.

The author acknowledges that within the scientific and medical fields, there are highly divergent views and opinions. This material is written expressly for the purpose of sharing educational information and scientific research gathered from the author's studies and experiences, healthcare professionals, scientists, nutritionists and informed health advocates.

None of the information contained in this book is intended to diagnose, prevent, treat, or cure any disease, nor to prescribe any of the techniques, materials, or concepts presented as a form of treatment for a medical condition.

Before starting any health, nutrition, or exercise-related practice, it is strongly recommended to obtain prior consent and advice from a licensed healthcare professional.

The author assumes no responsibility for the choices you make after reviewing the information contained in this document and consulting with a licensed healthcare professional.

None of the statements in this book have been evaluated by ANSES, the Food & Drug Administration (FDA), or the American Medical Association (AMA).

ACKNOWLEDGMENTS

Special thanks to Mark, Mira, Dr Raj and my husband Krasimir, who supported me during this transformation.

To my son Gabrillian, who I hope will one day read this book and understand that he is my greatest source of inspiration.

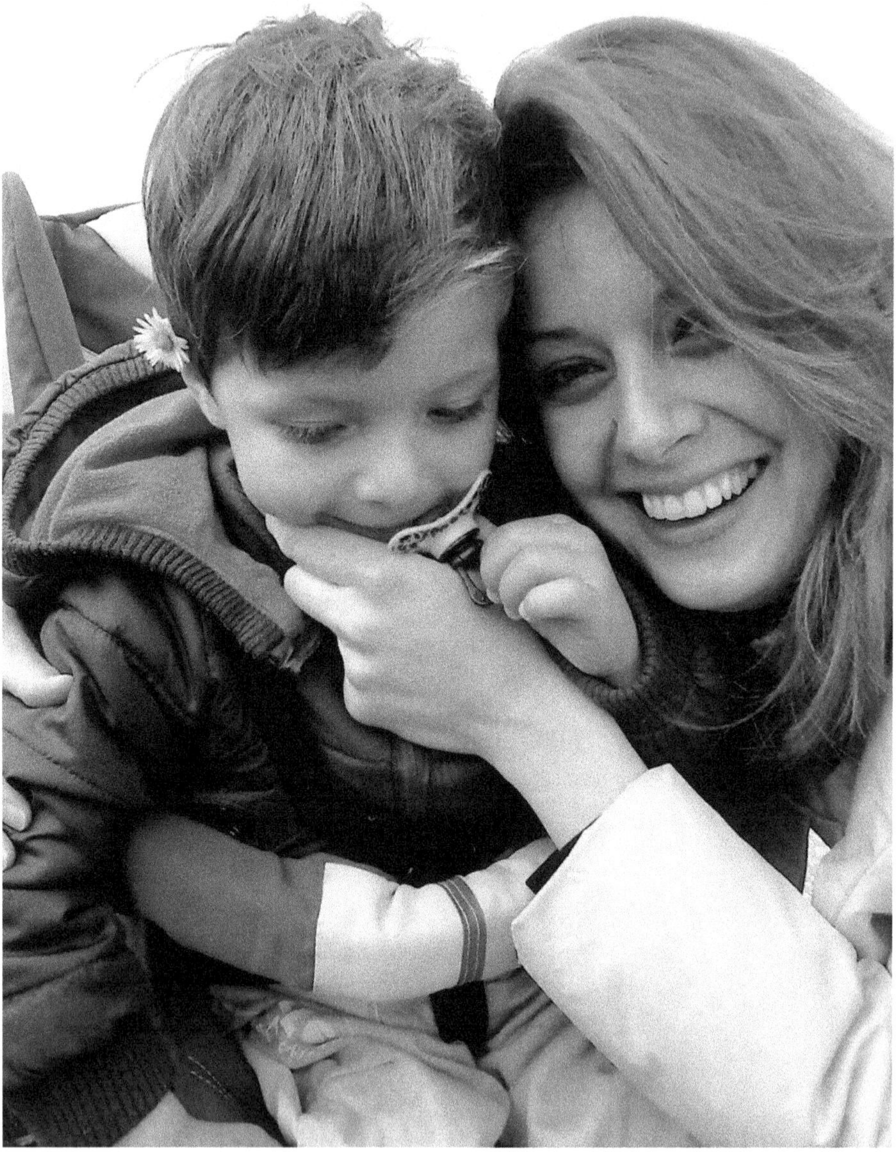

CONTENTS

PREFACE

This book tells the challenges that Gabrillian and his mother Clémentine experienced and ultimately conquered.
Is it possible to change a child's genetic anomaly—such as SMALED (spinal muscular atrophy)—to the point where nothing about their demeanour, physicality, or mentality shows any sign of it?

Where there is a strong desire, anything is possible.

But you will have to embark on a journey, you will have to change your identity and of course, transmit it to your child to the extent that none of your cells is infected by your lack of self-love, your lack of courage, your fear of the unknown or your resentment against what you may have perceived as unfair.

Every disease or imbalance begins with an emotion and a lack of self-love and you will have to find and transfer that love, balance and inner peace to your child, defying all the genetic ties that are woven into the dysfunctional fabric of a family.

Yes, this book will give you a specific diet for muscular dystrophy, detoxification tests and procedures, the manual and electronic techniques used, advice from experts, explanations of the primary causes of muscular dystrophy, but also the personal work of Gabrillian's mother both on herself and on Gabrillian to change her thoughts related to the imbalances of this disease.

And more than that, I hope you will be able to read in it the story of a person who long believed herself weak and powerless, to the point of letting others walk all over her, changing her destiny and that of her son, to that of someone who finds courage for her child and fights all her fears to transcribe her discoveries and guide other families to their own victory.

INTRODUCTION

***

November 25, 2017

Gabrillian and I made the journey from Cyprus to London to see Dr Raj and he was truly impressed with Gabrillian's progress. His gait is so different now—it seems like his feet and legs are more aligned with his body, compared to the previous vagus deformity where his feet used to point outward. Neurologists and kinesiologists had explained to me that it was the posture he had adopted, a sort of compensation due to his muscle atrophies in both quadriceps.

"Mom, look at me! Look at me!" Gabrillian shouts. Gabrillian and I were in Pinner Park, just 10 minutes from Northwood Hills station, where Dr Raj's clinic is located. It's late November and it's already quite cold in London, so we are wearing two pairs of pants and two sweaters.

It's around 4 o'clock in the afternoon and it's starting to get dark. Gabrillian is running on a muddy path along the park and I remind him to be careful not to slip, since we had left our travel backpack with spare clothes at Andrew's house, our host in London. I found this rental on Airbnb, right next to the building where Dr Raj works. Andrew and his wife have left us the key to their home because it's the second time we've stayed with them and we have established a good relationship.

I look at Gabrillian. He's walking slowly now and I remember how many times in the past he used to fall while walking. Before, he needed to run to avoid losing balance. Now he has only fallen once and I notice that when he loses balance, it's always after crossing his legs due to a lack of coordination.

Suzanna, his physiotherapist, told me during the last session, "It's not a lack of muscle strength; he's much stronger than before. Today, I placed a 0.5 kg weight on each of his legs and he walked on the treadmill for more than 10 minutes!"

Suzanna is also very enthusiastic about Gabrillian's physical performances and claims that he is more cooperative now. "Gabrillian, let's go, it's time," I remind him.

After the appointment, I promise to take him to a 'taverna.' It's a kind of restaurant offering traditional Cypriot cuisine and he has been talking about eating at a taverna during our evening walk for a month now.

I see him running towards me. He's now using his quadriceps muscles and bending his knees. Before, he didn't bend his knees or lift his thighs when walking, which created a lot of tension in his excessively tight knees.

After the appointment with Dr Raj, I found a Thai restaurant. I see a small sign on the door indicating that the house accommodates food allergies and that it is advisable to inquire.

"Hello. We would like to eat here. Also, my son has food intolerances, he can't eat gluten, dairy, sugar, is it possible?" I ask.

"Yes, of course. What would you like to eat?"

"Well, what do you suggest? What options are left?" I inquire. The waiter smiles, reviews the entire menu and looks at what he could offer us. After a few unsuccessful attempts, he decides to create a custom dish for Gabrillian: Shrimp with rice and eggs.

Gabrillian is excited; he's finally going to eat at a 'taverna', and they're bringing him a specially prepared meal.

"Mom, if I eat this, I'm going to get stronger. I'm going to grow and I'm going to run!"

***

December 2017

"How is Gabrillian?" I ask Vassilis, Gabrillian's father.

"He has a sore throat. I took him to the doctor and he said he has pharyngitis and gave him honey and lemon syrup," Vassilis replies. "Oh, great, because Gabrillian has citrus and sugar intolerances in all forms.!" I am boiling inside. How many times do I have to explain Gabrillian's special diet to him? "Hey, Chori, it's lemon and honey, it's good, it's full of vitamins!" Vassilis retorts.

"Fish is also good for health, but not if you have an allergy to iodine or if they are full of mercury," I counter.

"He doesn't have any allergies or intolerances, as you claim. I don't believe in what that doctor says. Besides, he's not a real doctor." Raj Bhachu from the Sai Nutrition Centre in London is a naturopath who uses a bio resonance device to perform tests for food allergies or toxicity. Bio resonance is based on cutting-edge molecular biology research. NASA discovered it.

"I don't believe in that nonsense," Vassilis interrupts.

I let him speak and then I remind him that he needs to bring Gabrillian to me at 6 o'clock tonight. There's no point in arguing further or trying to convince someone who already has their own theory. I remember that everything is a process and it's not up to me to change others; the results will speak for themselves.

CHAPTER 1
Gabrillian's birth

***

August 16, 2012

The caesarean section was scheduled for 7 in the morning. I hadn't slept all night.
"Aaaahhhh.!"
The new mother next to me had been screaming and complaining all night. It was one of those huge rooms with several beds side by side, separated only by a thick green curtain that provided some privacy.
I could hear everything and all possible scenarios went through my mind that night.
"The doctors stitched her up while she was awake; the epidural didn't last long enough," my partner Vassilis told me about the woman next door.
I was so stressed and scared.
"Is that even possible?!!" I exclaimed.
I remembered all the stories I had heard about Cypriot hospitals and I was far from reassured. Now I hear the sound of the hospital bed, the squeaking of the wheels. They come to get me to take me to the operating room. I'm already crying.
They take me to a white room for surgery.
"Please sit down!" the anaesthesiologist scolds.
How can I sit up straight? The nurses attacked me this morning to insert a urinary catheter! Another mistake! I'm at the end of my patience.
Finally, the anaesthesiologist—after numerous attempts—administers my injection and now they lay me on a metal bed and

restrain me. I start to panic. My heart is racing, I feel like I can't breathe and at the same time, I'm nauseous.

They begin the operation. Oh my God, when I look up, I realise that the lights are reflecting the scene, I can see the entire operation. Urrgh, I want to vomit.

They lift my baby into the air and I finally catch a glimpse of him, but I don't hear Gabrillian's cries. Finally, they bring him closer to my head and then "wahhhh..!"

I melt at the first sight of my precious son.

***

A few hours later

"Is something wrong? Why haven't they brought my baby to me? You would tell me if something was wrong, right?" I was completely panicked, Vassilis and his family reassure me.

"Gabrillian is perfect, he's under the lights."

It's 3:00 PM and I still haven't held my baby in my arms. At 5:00 PM, the nurses finally bring a little maternity bed with this tiny baby on it. I'm so happy and he already has his eyes open. A beautiful love story begins.

***

October 28, 2012

"I think my baby has a problem, his behaviour is not normal. He doesn't sleep during the day and all night, he cries incessantly." Dr Marios looks at me and I can see that his smile and certainty are starting to fade. It's the third time in a week that I've come to the Blue Cross clinic in Paphos, to explain my concerns.

"Are you ready?" he asks me, all excited about his new approach, handing me a new formula to try. It's probably powdered formula brought by one of those saleswomen who would interrupt us every time I see him, to offer new samples, new medicines. I don't feel any more reassured and I look at his desk, covered in pharmaceutical samples, my gaze vacant.

***

First trip to France. Gabrillian is 3 months old.

I couldn't bear to deal with doctors in Cyprus who send me back and forth without giving me any explanation and who see me as an overly concerned, annoying mother who invents stories! I was at my wit's end!

After discussing it with my parents, I made a decision. I prepare for my trip to France.

***

My mother looks at me, unable to believe how tired I am. I have travelled all day, alone with my 3-month-old baby. I finally arrive home in France. It's 11:00 PM. It's very cold in France compared to Cyprus. It's November.

"Go to bed right now! When was the last time you had a good night's sleep?"

***

One day later, we are at the "Mother and Child" hospital in Lyon. It's about an hour's drive from my parents' house because when we arrived my parents had noticed that Gabrillian was behaving strangely and the next day my mother insists that we take Gabrillian to the hospital - right away!

"You're lucky, Mrs. Ynna, you've come to the right place! I'm a paediatrician specialised in gastroenterology. Your son is suffering from oesophagitis. It's inflammation of the oesophagus, the throat. I'll prescribe him Inexium, which is a medication that doctors usually prescribe for stomach ulcers. At low doses, it will work for him and he should be healed in about 8 days. I'll also write a letter to one of my colleagues; she's an allergist. It would be advisable to check whether the little one has a dairy allergy." I'm so relieved. Maybe now Gabrillian will finally stop crying day and night.

Later, we went to the paediatrician's colleague. However, she didn't find a lactose allergy and she mentioned that there might be a possibility that the test wouldn't show intolerances. She wants to prescribe a special lactose-free milk, but she doesn't know if I'll be able to find it in Cyprus and she explains that the price of this milk is so high that to afford it, I might eventually have to "survive on potatoes".

***

February 2013

A few months ago, we decided to move to France. We packed up everything, our furniture, our clothes. It was so exhausting; I thought the move would never end.

Today was the last step before our new life in another country, my country, with my family. I'm excited but also very sad.

Vassilis stops the car in front of his parents' house. It's very early in the morning. His mother and father come out to the car.

Gabrillian is half asleep in the back seat. My heart breaks when I watch them try, in vain, to hold back their tears.

The neighbour also comes to bid us farewell; she doesn't hide her sorrow and bursts into floods of tears.

Vassilis's brother sits in front. He will come with us to Larnaca and drive the car back. Vassilis starts the car. I look through the rear windshield. Gabrillian's grandparents wave goodbye to us and quickly go back inside.

I know they'll start crying as soon as they close the door.

***

May 2013

"Please, can you stop with those damn movies, go see my sister and learn French so that you can find a job?"

I look at Vassilis. He's sprawled out on the bed, staring at his computer screen. The room is in complete disarray. I can't take it anymore.

I wonder if it was a mistake to move to France so quickly. Vassilis can't even have a simple conversation in French and doesn't seem interested in learning the language.

I understand that he's depressed. It's the first time he's left his country, except for a week spent in England. He had hated life there and couldn't wait to get back to Cyprus.

Living in France was a choice we made together. He said, "I can do it because you also decided to leave your country to be with me." I didn't know it would be so hard for him. It's been two months now since we've been living in my parents' house and not a day goes by without me arguing with my parents or with Vassilis.

Then one day, out of the blue, Vassilis announces "My sister is getting married, I'm going back to Cyprus,"

"How? We don't have the money for that! We don’t have the money for anything! " I say.

"My father will pay for my ticket."

"But we just found you a job interview in Lyon next week!" "I won't stay just for an interview! I'm going to Cyprus." He snaps.

***

"Mom, I'm going to Martine's to give her a massage. Gabrillian is sleeping! I'll be back in about two hours."

"It's okay, Clémentine, but don't take too long because I can't do anything with Gabrillian if he fusses and I'm tired."

It's been a month now since Vassilis went to Cyprus. He has ended up staying there to try to find a job. I stayed at my parents' house with Gabrillian. I give massages to my mom's friends and friends of friends to make some money.

Gabrillian no longer has acid reflux, that has calmed down significantly with the Inexium and that, as well as sitting upright and eating solid food, has helped him a lot.

Vassilis calls us every other night. In general, we end up arguing. One night, I break down. We're on the verge of breaking up. I don't want to go back to Cyprus anymore.

A few days later, I go to pick up Vassilis at St Exupéry Airport. It's about a 45-minute drive from my place. I decide to give him another chance and forget everything but a few weeks later, I receive two job offers in Cyprus and Vassilis begs me to come back.

***

Return to Cyprus, February 2014

"Gabrillian, come here! Come here my sweetheart," I call to my son.
Gabrillian is now 18 months old. He can stand, but constantly falls. It's as if he has no balance.

He now comes towards me, holding onto the living room table to keep his balance.
Since Gabrillian is my first child, I have no experience with the milestones for when a child is supposed to walk, so I'm not worried. Nevertheless, my mother and I decide to take Gabrillian to the orthopaedist.

She examines Gabrillian's feet and confirms that he walks on the sides of his feet and on his heels.

"Don't worry. Some children don't walk until they're 2 years old," the orthopaedist tells me.

So, as she advised, I don't worry.

***

A Myopathy?

One day, Gabrillian's Cypriot grandmother decides to take him to an orthopaedic surgeon who was visiting Cyprus to offer his services. Gabrillian is now two years old and still falls a lot when he walks.

He has adopted a way of walking with a certain waddle that Dr Ferrero, the paediatric director of the Bourgoin hospital in France, will later call "a duck waddle."

The orthopaedist sends us directly to Dr Paula Nicolaidis, a paediatric neurologist in Limassol.

***

"Gabrillian, come here right now!"

I can't take chasing after Gabrillian anymore. We have waited for half an hour in the waiting room and now he's fed up and is hiding under the doctor's desk.

"You're lucky to have a son like that," she says with a smile and I wonder if she's mocking me. But she seems sincere.

Dr Paula talks to me about ‘muscle weakness,’ ‘weak lower limbs,’ ‘hypotonia’.

I'm still not worried; to me, muscle weakness is a weakness that can easily be strengthened with some kinesiology, appropriate exercises and maybe some swimming.

Then Dr Paula hands me a medical referral letter for an EMG at the American Hospital in Nicosia.

***

What is an electromyogram?

I find myself in a difficult situation again.

The doctor asks me to distract Gabrillian with a book and Vassilis has to hold his hands. What are they going to do to him?

I see the doctor approaching Gabrillian's leg with a large needle. Another person helps hold his thigh.

I see Gabrillian's eyes turn toward the needle. He screams!

I try to distract him, to tell him it'll be over soon, that it will be quick. The doctor starts sending an electric shock into his leg. Gabrillian wails, screaming louder. I feel so helpless, I don't know what to do to calm him.

I realise they don't really have any experience with children. I know I need to regain my composure because if I am stressed, Gabrillian will sense it and it certainly won't help.

"Remove that damn thing from my son's leg right now!" Vassilis is angry.

Suddenly, Vassilis explodes and removes the needle himself, cursing the doctors. He grabs Gabrillian by the hand and we are out of the facility!

Gabrillian was terrified by this experience. He told everyone he met after that, "the doctor gave me a shot!"

After this experience, we decide that all tests, examinations, MRI's, muscle biopsies, etc., would be done in France.

***

Trip to France, November 2014

My sister managed to get an appointment with Dr Ferrero, the paediatric director of the Bourgoin hospital.

The paediatrician observes Gabrillian. He throws toys to the other side of the room and asks my son to pick them up and bring them back to him. He observes how Gabrillian walks, bends down and stands up. In fact, Gabrillian bends down with difficulty and needs to rest his hands on his knees to stand up.

Dr Ferrero checks for knee and ankle reflexes that he does not find and then asks Gabrillian to reach for an object up high. Gabrillian can't reach it because he cannot stand on tip toes. He can't jump. Later, Dr Ferrero will note in his report to his colleague Dr Manel, a paediatric neurologist at the Lyon hospital:

"I examined little Gabrillian. his gait resembles that of a duck. He has a positive Gower sign".

At the end of the session, I try to learn more about the decision to send us to a paediatric neurologist because Dr Ferrero had not given me his opinion.

"Could we consider expediting the procedures and request an urgent consultation, given that we are returning to Cyprus in a few days?" I ask.

"There's no urgency in Gabrillian's case, but I would advise you to seek help immediately. Parents often need psychological support." He says his expression serious.

The paediatrician's voice softens. I feel like I'm in a bad dream. I don't understand. Is Gabrillian's case so severe? What is it, why would we need psychological help?

The doctor shakes his head. He doesn't know; he can't make a diagnosis. But, from the softening of his voice and the compassion in his glance, I understand that Gabrillian's health is of grave concern and taking medication or appropriate therapy is not going to solve the problem.

My mother cries and talks to the doctor.

It's as if a movie is playing out before my eyes and I have no control of what is happening. In fact, I'm not even part of the scene anymore. I'm there without being there.

The doctor says, "Do you have any questions, madam?"

"Sorry. um, no, I don't have any questions." I mumble. Actually I have thousands but I know that he doesn't have the answers.

***

We finally get an appointment with Dr Manel to redo the EMG. My parents pay for Gabrillian and me to travel because financially, we can't afford to travel to France every few months for his exams.

"Look, Gabrillian!" I am trying to distract my son but Gabrillian is not happy at all, I feel he is about to explode.

Dr Manel's assistant hands a green teddy bear to Gabrillian. She puts a mask on his face and explains what's going to happen. She shows him the needle and places it on his hand so he can feel it. I realise it's more like an electrode.

"You see, it's a bit cold," the assistant says. "Dr Manel will send a small current; it will feel like a little sting."

Thankfully, Gabrillian starts to calm down. The gas flowing into his mask is relaxing him.

Dr Manel begins the procedure. When she sends the electric shock, Gabrillian flinches, he doesn't like it and he complains. Dr Manel enters different data into her computer but soon Gabrillian can't take it anymore. We have to stop the procedure.

I ask her what she thinks. Does she have any similar cases? My mother asks if he has Duchenne's disease. She replies that he doesn't. She says she leans toward a diagnosis of Spinal Muscular Atrophy (SMA) and says she will research types I and III. She also tells me it's possible that Gabrillian might end up with only a slight waddle. That reassures me.

In the car, even though the doctors recommend not doing it, I ask my mother for her phone to look up what SMA type I and III are on the internet.

I read a few words.

I collapse.

***

On January 1, 2015, eleven months after our return to Cyprus, I separate from Gabrillian's father. Gabrillian is two and a half years old. I tend to avoid conflicts, but I realised that it was no longer possible to continue. The arguments were constant.

The bad news about Gabrillian's health along with Vassilis not wanting to accept the reality that his son had a problem, hadn't helped either. Vassilis is a good-hearted person and loves his son very much, but I couldn't reconcile myself with this mentality. He had changed since I gave birth to Gabrillian and so had I, undoubtedly.

I had understood that in Cyprus, the women of the house didn't have much say in child-rearing. And yet, how many times had he left me alone with Gabrillian, in favour of spending time with his friends?

I also struggled to accept that Vassilis's mother takes such ownership of Gabrillian. Whenever Gabrillian cries, she takes him from my arms to comfort him. It was certainly well-intentioned, to relieve me of my fatigue, but I always had this lump in my throat, was she telling me that I wasn't capable of taking care of my own son?

As I began to distance myself, Vassilis senses it and becomes increasingly jealous. One night, he had been drinking and got too carried away with me, while Gabrillian cried. I knew then that I couldn't go on like this and so I asked Vassilis to leave. At first, he wanted to take Gabrillian with him and we argued until I was exhausted. Finally, Vassilis took his car and left. He felt it was the end. I moved to an apartment a few minutes from Kouklia, Gabrillian's grandparents' village. I was devastated. Every morning, while I took Gabrillian to school, I cried. Vassilis's mother had come to apologise and told me it was her fault, that she hadn't raised her son properly. Vassilis's father, on the other hand, would barely nod in greeting.

***

"Gabrillian, come on!"

It's the same drama every time! I've come to pick up Gabrillian from his grandparents' house. Every evening after work, I go to get him and always, he doesn't want to come with me. There he goes, crying again. "Oxi! Oxi! (no, no), sometimes he even ends up rolling on the floor.

I observe his way of walking. He can't take two steps without falling. He falls to the ground as soon as I touch him. Thoughts rush through my head. How am I going to deal with Gabrillian? I remember Vassilis's father's face and I am sure they all hate me in this family. Gabrillian doesn't want to stay with me; he's bored with me. I'm not a good mother and clearly, they think I don't know how to take care of my son.

As I recall the scene when Gabrillian cries and screams that he doesn't want to come with me, I feel anger and resentment. Everything wells up. I feel shame, embarrassment and guilt. All of this is my fault. In that moment, I feel very alone. I had argued with my own family in France and had stopped calling them. As if that wasn't enough, old family stories resurfaced and I resented them. They had meddled too much in my relationship with Vassilis. I do have friends, but in recent years, I had neglected them to be with the friends I shared with Vassilis whom I can tell are on his side or will try to patch things up.

Gabrillian was very unhappy with this situation. He kept asking me why we had separated and said that he missed his daddy. I also noticed that his gait had worsened.

It felt like my whole world had collapsed. I didn't know what to do anymore. I went from anger to hope and from sadness to frustration.

I was ready to explode at any moment.

CHAPTER 2
First, Changing My Mindset

***

The wind is changing.

One day, I make a decision that will change my entire life. About six months earlier, I had met Mira at my job as a masseuse at the Aphrodite Hills Intercontinental Hotel. Mira is a hypnotherapist. She explains to me and my colleagues that the subconscious mind governs over 80% of our actions. I'm intrigued.

Mira is willing to offer us a free session! However, my colleagues are sceptical. "It's satanic, it's evil, it brainwashes you!" They are very religious in Cyprus.

At the time, I wasn't the type of person to take risks and I relied a lot on others' opinions. I let the opportunity pass.

I met Mira a couple more times and after reading Paulo Coelho's book, "The Alchemist," I see it as a sign.

This book was a revelation to me. The constant quest to find happiness is the reason we are here. We search everywhere for a magical solution, not realising that the solution is already inside us.

I was sitting on my couch in front of my computer, looking for motivating music because I felt lonely and depressed and then, this quote by author Viktor Frankl appeared on my screen:

"When we are no longer able to change a situation, we are challenged to change ourselves!"

And then - it clicked!

***

How many times have I felt this emotion of helplessness, loneliness, abandonment?

A vision appears in my mind, like a spiral, a repetition of events that generates the same emotions.

I remember the day I was told that my mom had passed away. I was 5 years old and I didn't want to believe it. I remember running through our big house, searching every room for my mom. When I reached her room with its closed shutters and the musty smell, I knew then it was true. I went back downstairs and found my father in tears. I felt lost. I had a lump in my throat and felt sick.

And then, I felt abandoned.

"Your sisters and you will stay with Aunt Sylvie and Uncle Didier and I will come back to get you," my dad had told us. When he returned from his trips, he always brought us something, a doll, toys, but what I looked forward to the most was one of his Marlboro cigarette packs which, when I gently flipped open the lid revealed – ladybugs! They say ladybugs are the good Lord's creatures. We would go into the garden, and with the release of each ladybug, I would send messages to my mom in heaven, as they had shown me, telling me that my mum was now in the sky.

Then, my dad had to leave again and this time we had to stay with Aunt Nicole and my godfather Jean Louis.

I missed my dad; I felt so abandoned again. And then one day, when he came to pick us up, he wanted to introduce us to our "new mom." Her name was Corinne; she already had three daughters and she was going to live with us. I wasn't ready for this, or for her to ask me to call her "mom" - I already had a mom!

Fanny, my half-sister and me often fought, maybe because we were almost the same age and I often felt that she wanted to dominate me.

When we sat at the table, I always had a knot in my stomach. What would happen this time? Would I end up in my room because I wouldn't accept the authority of my new mom?

Would Fanny and I fight, again? Would I open my mouth and hear my sisters laugh at me? Would my dad have that desperate look on his face? I think he was ashamed of me. Once again, I felt very alone.

I grew up, still with that knot in my stomach when I was invited to a meal or a party, anywhere with lots of people. I waited for the moment when, unable to stop myself, I would say something inappropriate or do something clumsy. There would always be that moment when I would make a fool of myself and want to disappear.

Little by little, I cultivated the art of being invisible. Only at high school, did I get all the attention - my teachers even thought I was very intelligent! Sometimes I wondered how I could be so popular at school and so miserable at home.

All these experiences triggered the same emotions again and again, repeating experiences that made me feel the same emotions, like a vicious cycle.

I was determined and ready to do anything to change that.

***

I decide to call Mira for a hypnotherapy session.

"Hello, it's Clementine. I want to have a hypnosis session. When do you think you would have some free time for me?" It's strange. For the first time, I didn't try to justify myself and made an instant decision without thinking too much about it. This was new and I realised that making a decision without consulting my mother, my sisters, or getting my friends' opinions was exhilarating! I had taken a risk! And also, I had followed my instinct. My intuition had become my new companion and comrade.

I was far from realising how many new initiatives and risks I would take after this first simple decision or how addicted I would become to this new way of thinking and living. Mira asks me where I am and if I can make it in half an hour.

I can and I do!

I am in front of the Holistic Centre in Paphos, where Mira works as a freelancer. It's a grey day. We are in February.

Mira arrives. I follow her. We climb a small stone staircase, she pushes a door open and we enter a room dominated by purple. She suggests I sit down and we begin the session.

She has just completed a new program called 'releasing breathing techniques.' She asks me if I would like to try it. This technique involves holding your breath when you make affirmations because this way, the subconscious is drawn to the surface. This works because our conscious brain has no oxygen supply and if it feels in danger the subconscious takes control, to ensure survival. The advantage is that the subconscious doesn't know if what you're affirming is true or false, a dream or reality. You can tell it whatever you want, or rather, whatever you wish for. You can recreate your story by changing scenes and in doing so, react completely differently to the same situation.

***

"When the student is ready, the master appears."

I had already heard of this, although I still had doubts. But it was worth a try. After all, what did I have to lose?

***

"What is the reason for your visit? What do you expect from this session?" Mira asks.

"I don't really know." I burst into tears.

"I don't know anymore. As I explained to you before, I have separated from my ex and although I know it's a good decision, I can't handle it, with Gabrillian, my job...." I list all my problems. After listening to me carefully, Mira hands me a piece of paper and asks me to write down everything that bothers me about others, the changes I would like to make, etc.

I take several deep breaths and over about twenty minutes Mira recites many affirmations starting with "I now remove and release all emotional blocks, both positive and negative."

She will explain to me later that this is a way of eliminating and replacing all thoughts and emotional blocks we wish to change. Indeed, all our experiences and even those of our parents are linked to our emotions.

Once this phase is over, I feel completely drained. Afterwards, Mira continues with the phase she calls "filling".

"I am now so grateful and happy that...."

After that, I feel like my diaphragm relaxes and my solar plexus radiates. I feel light, full of self-confidence and I have a strange sense of gratitude for everything around me. If, before, I only saw the bad and the drama in my situation, I can now see heroism in it, affirm my choices and decisions and something deep inside me tells me that the adventure is just beginning.

I move forward with a self-confidence that was previously unknown to me. I have the taste of victory on my tongue. Mira suggests that I participate in a program that will start the following month, to improve each attendee's confidence. I've already made up my mind. I'm going to do it!

***

"Good evening, everyone."

Mira starts the session.

It's been three months now since I started this program and even though I still hesitate to speak and describe my various experiences with the group, I already feel different. I have changed most of the relationships I had before I started the program but not without effort. Every morning and every evening in my car, I practice "releasing" and repeat the affirmations I want to manifest. For example, for my relationship with Vassilis's parents, I repeat, "I now release all resentment and guilt towards Gabrillian's grandparents."

I practice releasing for my son as well! His tantrums don't work on me anymore because now I release all the guilt and choose responsibility. I constantly affirm that I am a good mother because I take care of him; I choose to spend quality time with my son, even if it's only twenty minutes a day when I can focus solely on him.

And it works! Gabrillian is already calmer and more stable. He doesn't cry every time I pick him up from Vassilis's anymore and lately Gabrillian's tantrums no longer make his sneaky grandfather smile and don't irritate me either.

I also started writing in my "success journal" where I summarise all the successes of my day, my discoveries, my inspirations, the wisdom and the lessons I draw from different experiences. And soon, I find my vocabulary is changing. Instead of 'problems,' I now see challenges and opportunities.

I write down my wildest aspirations and I begin planning Gabrillian's healing although I didn't really know how to achieve it. When Mira told me to write down the logical steps, I wrote, "My son receives the best educational and medical support and fantastic financial support".

I could not have known that this is exactly what would happen! Very quickly, my life completely changed. I went from being a lost single mother to an organised and focused woman, determined to help her child.

"You've changed. It's like day and night!" My family in France couldn't believe the change in me.

Every time I faced a 'challenge,' I could now see the positive side and understand the lessons that came with it. I distanced myself from events and began to act instead of reacting.

I started spending more time with Gabrillian, playing games together, taking him to various playgrounds. He became much more stable and it was a joy to see him happy and laughing.

And because one happiness never comes alone, I have also attracted a new companion into my life, Krasimir.

Gabrillian and Krasimir took their time to 'get to know each other,' but gradually, they became friends and developed a mutual respect.

The stages of my mindset change and to summarise, this is how I did it;

- ***Making my own decisions/trusting my own guidance and intuition***
- ***Believing in myself despite any risk***
- ***'Releasing breathing' technique***
- ***'Releasing emotion' Sedona technique***
- ***Listening to a hypnosis audiobook every evening***
- ***Writing in my 'Success Journal' every night***
- ***Writing down my aspirations and the first logical steps I need to take.***

CHAPTER 3
New Discoveries

***

April 24, 2015

I met Mark at Aphrodite Hills in Cyprus, where he lives. He has a publishing house in London and he has published dozens of books on alternative medicine. He is particularly interested in how people can heal themselves naturally, without drugs or surgical interventions, by improving their nutrition and lifestyle.

One day, knowing that I was particularly distraught following the prognosis I had been given by Gabrillian's doctor, he sent me an email about heavy metal detoxification, its impact on the body and the consequences of heavy metal poisoning, one of which is malnutrition.
"Hello Clémentine, how are you? Listen, I'm writing a book about health and during my research, I came across some surprising information that I'm sure could help Gabrillian. Now, you can tell me that I don't know anything about Gabrillian's disease, but I would really like you to take a look at what I found." He said, the enthusiasm in his voice obvious.

"The first thing I want you to understand, Clémentine, is that in 99% of cases, there will be a natural solution to heal a person, regardless of their health problem. You must absolutely keep hold of hope for Gabrillian and you must conduct intensive research to discover the root cause of his illness. You find that and the battle is already half-won!

The name of a disease—such as 'Muscular Dystrophy'—is just a label attached to the condition by a doctor, a label placed on a collection of symptoms. What does 'Muscular Dystrophy' really mean? Well, the word 'dystrophy' comes from Greek—'trophi' means 'nutrition,' 'feeding,' 'growth'; 'dys' is the root of the word 'difficult' (dyskolo) or 'problematic, bad, abnormal.'"

"In other words, 'Muscular Dystrophy' simply means 'muscle malnutrition,' 'a lack of nutrition to the muscles,' 'nutrition that reaches the muscles with difficulty,' 'difficult muscle growth,' or simply **'the nutrition of muscle tissues is problematic or not working well!'**"

Mark continued his explanation.

"The word 'Amyotrophy' also comes from Greek—actually, from three Greek words. 'Myo,' derived from the ancient Greek μῦς ('mys,' which means muscle); τροφή ('trophi,' meaning food, growth); and α- (a privative prefix) which means 'non' or 'none.' So, the word 'a-amyotrophy' simply means **a lack of muscle growth or nutrition!**"

This discovery was a great revelation for me. A moment of enlightenment!
Paradoxically, all the labels and medical jargon had distanced me from the source, the root cause of my son's health problem. These scientific terms actually blocked my understanding and any search for measures to solve this problem.

When I understood the root of the words and their deep meaning, a change began to occur in my thinking. Now, I was dealing with something I understood, something I could address. I realised the potential of my son's own healing abilities and I regained my power, as a mother, to guide him through this process.
So, as Mark suggested, I started asking better questions.

"To overcome muscular dystrophy, we must first discover why nutrition is not reaching Gabrillian's muscles, secondly, we need to know how to achieve much higher levels of nutrition and thirdly, to ensure that these nutrients reach his muscles most effectively."

Mark continued to send me information that he had discovered about muscular dystrophy:

> **Clue #1: Muscular dystrophy could be caused by mercury poisoning.** A man called Ken Presner cured himself of multiple sclerosis (MS) and Crohn's disease by detoxifying himself of mercury and other heavy metals. In his book Against All Odds, Presner says:
>
> "Nearly 100% of the hundreds of cases of multiple sclerosis that I have seen over the past 18 years, have a history of mercury amalgam fillings. It is actually a very rare case of MS where there are no mercury amalgam fillings in the patient's history, or in their mother's history. Mercury crosses the placenta and is up to twice as concentrated in the foetus as in the mother. Hence suspicion around autism, cerebral palsy, mental retardation, ADD, MD (muscular dystrophy) bolstered by the 2008 lawsuit against the FDA by Moms Against Mercury concerning autistic children." 'You may have heard of children with ADHD (attention deficit disorder), autism, mental retardation, muscular dystrophy, cerebral palsy and type I diabetes. Dental mercury crosses the placenta and poisons the brain and other organs and systems of the developing foetus. Incredibly, mercury is often measured at double the mercury levels in the foetus compared to the mother. Dental mercury particularly targets the brain. It also attacks all the glands of the endocrine system, including the thyroid gland and the pancreas.' 'The sad truth is that for decades, millions of people have suffered and died from mercury poisoning hidden behind

various other disease names: autism, attention deficit disorder (ADHD), mental retardation, MD (muscular dystrophy), cerebral palsy, multiple sclerosis, Alzheimer's disease, Parkinson's disease, Lou Gehrig's disease (ALS) and Lupus.'

Children without mercury fillings can be autistic or suffer from other serious neurological problems like ADHD (attention deficit disorder). But they are still toxic from mercury. Mercury can escape from the mother's fillings, cross the placenta and end up in the brain of the unborn child. Mercury is also in breast milk. Dental mercury is so powerful that autism, ADHD, mental retardation, MD (muscular dystrophy) and cerebral palsy can result from the mother's 'silver fillings'. These facts are well documented.'

(Source: Against All Odds, by Ken Presner)

A few days later, Mark sends me additional information.

"Clémentine, I sent an email to Ken Presner about Gabrillian's muscular dystrophy. He responded, *'I haven't had a case of muscular dystrophy yet. But detoxifying toxic children is the way to go, in my opinion.'*"

"*I don't exactly know how mercury poisoning can interfere with nutrition reaching the muscles—it could be due to the damage caused by mercury to the intestines. Dental amalgams, pesticides or vaccines (sources of heavy metals) could be the cause. In any case, I think it's vital for Gabrillian to be tested for heavy metals (blood, urine and hair analysis)*."

Mark added the following information to his email:

Clue #2: Muscular dystrophy could be caused by a lack of selenium and other minerals. Naturopath Joel Wallach writes:

"MUSCULAR DYSTROPHY is another crime against the human population by 'orthodox' doctors for monetary reasons. If the whole truth were shared with the public, muscular dystrophy would be entirely preventable, but an entire medical speciality would be annihilated, in the process!

Look at the veterinary industry where muscle is 'king' (i.e., pork chops, beef steaks, lamb chops, roasts, ground beef, chicken, turkey, etc.) In animals, muscular dystrophy has been eradicated! A farmer with 100 cows can expect 100 conceptions, 100 live births, 100 normal calves and 100 calves raised to market or breeding age. How is it that animals are better treated and have better outcomes than humans? Prevention is vital when it comes to Muscular Dystrophy. "The levels of selenium in preconception women are important for maintaining pregnancy as well as preventing muscular dystrophy in all its forms (i.e., Duchenne, Erb scapulohumeral myopathy, Leyden-Moebius pelvi-femoral, Landouzy-Dejerine, Becker and Gowers), which are artificial classifications of muscular dystrophy by the initially affected muscle groups. Keshan disease (cardiac muscular dystrophy), which is also caused by selenium deficiency, should be added to the list of muscular dystrophies."

"In the veterinary profession, muscular dystrophy ('White Muscle Disease') has been eliminated using selenium in pregnant animals and in rapidly growing prepubertal animals. In addition to manifest selenium deficiencies in the diet, changes in the type of celiac disease in the small intestine caused by food allergies are a frequent cause of tissue selenium deficiencies. Symptoms of muscular dystrophy can begin with weakness, scoliosis (curvature of the spine) and hypertrophy of certain muscle groups (e.g., calves, trapezius, etc.) to compensate for the loss of strength in synergistic muscle groups. A muscle biopsy is usually performed by a neurologist to establish the diagnosis of muscular dystrophy. If selenium and vitamin E were to be administered IM or IV at the very first onset of symptoms, the disease would be stopped or perhaps even 'cured.' Orthodox doctors resort to prednisone and surgery. It would be much healthier to seek help from a veterinarian!" (Source: "Let's Play Doctor" by Joel Wallach)

Clue #3: Muscular dystrophy and nutritional therapy - CoQ10 therapy, Vitamin E, Selenium, Lecithin, etc.

"During our son's last visit to the paediatrician, the doctor was completely amazed at how well he was doing. He shows no signs of the typical muscular dystrophy that she expected to see, based on her experience with conventional medicine."

"I was diagnosed with a form of FSHD muscular dystrophy a few years ago and heard the typical comment - 'there is no known cure' - from the orthopaedist, neurosurgeon and my family doctor. I accepted the situation but continued to hope for some development in the treatment of the disease. I came across your website and read the article on muscular dystrophy. For the first time in years, I felt encouraged and began trying a combination of the elements listed in the article. I noticed an immediate increase in my energy levels, which was good in itself, but then recently, the 'incredible' happened when my wife and I noticed an increase in the size of the calf muscle in my left leg (without exercise). It was very obvious. I continue with the vitamins and supplements with impatient anticipation."

"Everyone knows what muscles are and when they don't work, the weakness, fragility and helplessness of a young child with muscular dystrophy make for a poignant image and a tearful telethon. 'There is no treatment. There is no specific therapy,' says the Merck Manual. Such autocratic and desperate statements should not be considered the last word until we have sufficiently assessed maternal and foetal malnutrition as a possible fundamental cause of muscular dystrophy. The good news (to be examined in more detail below) is that if a nutrient deficiency can cause a disease, nutritional therapy can improve or even cure that disease."

"Does malnutrition cause muscular dystrophy? The short answer is yes. 'Dystrophy: 1. Defective nutrition. 2. Any disorder caused by defective nutrition.' (Definition in the American Heritage Dictionary of the English Language, p 407.)"

"Like CoQ10, vitamin E is an antioxidant. There is a long history of scientific suspicion, as yet largely untested, that antioxidants are of unusual benefit to people with muscular dystrophy." American chemist Linus Pauling (Nobel Prize in Chemistry in 1954 and Nobel Peace Prize in 1962) wrote about muscular dystrophy, both experimental and hereditary, in his book "How to Live Longer and Feel Better":

"It has been recognised for more than fifty years that a low intake of vitamin E causes muscular dystrophy, a disorder of the skeletal muscles characterised by weakness similar to that caused by a deficiency of vitamin C (studies on vitamin E and muscular dystrophies were discussed by Pappenheimer in 1948). Several types of hereditary muscular dystrophies are known. For most of them, their nature is not completely understood and no specific therapy is recommended for them. Severe myasthenia is treated with cholinesterase inhibitors, corticosteroids and surgical removal of the thymus. Medical authorities do not mention the possible value of vitamins in controlling muscular dystrophies. The evidence of the involvement of vitamin E and vitamin C as well as B6 and other vitamins in muscle function suggests that optimal intakes of these nutrients should be helpful to patients. As far as I know, no comprehensive study of increased vitamin E intake for patients with hereditary muscular dystrophy has been reported."

"Except for the CoQ10 studies referenced above, unfortunately Dr Pauling's statement from 20 years ago still holds up well. I found a few studies, one with 15 patients using vitamin E and selenium reporting 'minimal' benefits and another with 16 patients showing 'mild' benefit. I think they would have obtained much better results if they had used larger doses of selenium, much larger doses of vitamin E and only vitamin E in its natural form."

"Then there was a study, using 600 mg of vitamin E and a high amount of selenium (4,000 mcg of Na2SeO3), which achieved very good results in the five patients studied. All improved their grip strength, two normalised their gait, two others can now sit on their heels and stand up. One patient can now walk on tiptoes, one can now get up from a lying position on the floor without using a chair and two patients improved their physical ability. No side effects were observed. This is, at the very least, truly encouraging."

"Don't forget: 'Dystrophy' means 'malnutrition.' There is no drug that corrects malnutrition and ***there never will be***.

Agronomists know this. You will have little difficulty finding research studies on the role of selenium or vitamin E in the prevention of muscular dystrophies in chickens, cattle, calves, sheep or lambs. What works with calves should, in my opinion, reasonably also apply to humans."

"However, despite the long and costly history of human muscular dystrophy research, only a very small part has involved vitamins and that research was done some time ago. In the third edition of 'The Vitamins in Medicine,' Bicknell and Prescott provide a comprehensive review of the literature on pages 612-619 and 635-641. There is ample evidence that the disease is an inability of muscle tissue to effectively use vitamin E. I give you the following quote: 'The particular muscle degeneration of muscular dystrophy that can be produced in animals is caused and is only caused by a lack of vitamin E. Human muscular dystrophy similarly shows the same particular degeneration. The key to the treatment of muscular dystrophy is vitamin E.' (See: Rabinovitch R et al (1951))." "Muscular dystrophy is described as easier to cure in children and even easier with added B and C vitamins (p 644). We have ignored the evidence and doctors continue to tell patients that Muscular Dystrophy is incurable."

I was frozen in place, stunned. I could hardly believe it, but this was stronger than me. I felt a glimmer of hope rising in me. Was it possible that a dietary deficiency was the cause of Gabrillian's disease? And was it possible to turn the tide by changing his diet?

I had just completed a seminar on Ayurvedic medicine and Sachin, the instructor, was talking about the importance of digestion. He explained that a malfunction of digestion leads to metabolic errors and creates toxins. *It all starts with digestion*. Sachin emphasised, 'Once sleep and digestion are restored, you are already 50% cured.'

These words resonate with me. If we want better answers, we must ask better questions.

In summary New questions:

- **Is Muscular Dystrophy heavy metal poisoning?**
- **Is malnutrition an indirect consequence of heavy metal poisoning?**
- **Does poor digestion lead to metabolic errors such as enzyme or amino acid deficiencies?**

Once the restoration of good digestion and sleep is in place, is the person 50% cured?"

CHAPTER 4

A visit to Doctor Georgiou at the Da Vinci Holistic Centre

***

November 2016

Sometime later, Mark suggests that I publish a book about Muscular Dystrophy. He would like to highlight Gabrillian's case as an example that will inspire families with children suffering from this disease. He offers to pay for all the consultations, supplements etc.

"What do you think, Clementine?" Mark asks me.

I stammer, "Uh, yes, of course! That would be great!"

This was unexpected, nothing short of a miracle!

And here we are, embarking on a new adventure. Gabrillian would be able to benefit from much more medical support than I had ever hoped for or imagined.

Mark asked me to make appointments with two doctors. One of them was in Cyprus, Dr George Georgiou.

***

Dr Georgiou had opened an holistic centre, the Da Vinci Centre in Larnaca. He is a naturopath specialising in heavy metal detoxification and candidiasis.

"Gabrillian, sit down! Gabrillian, no! Don't go outside! Wait! Gabrillian!!" I run out of the office to catch up with my son. There is a birdcage in the holistic centre's garden that caught Gabrillian's attention. I soften as I see him talking to the birds. He has always loved animals since he was little. Also, we have just completed a long journey. It takes about an hour and a half to drive between Pissouri and Larnaca. It's a long journey for a hyperactive little boy like Gabrillian!

I decide he is probably better left outside.

Gabrillian brought his own toys, Playmobil toys and plastic animals. He likes to play with them, all at once. They fight, they attack each other. I have tried to play with him and I must say I was a bit lost - his stories made no sense to me! Eventually, he told me he preferred to play alone and I noticed that this is often the case at school too; he plays by himself.

"Miss Ynna, Gabrillian, please come in, the doctor will see you now," calls the receptionist.

***

"So, tell me, what brings you here? Tell me more about Gabrillian's case," Dr Georgiou says.

"Gabrillian has, well, it's not certain, they are still researching but the doctors have said that he has muscle atrophy in both quadriceps. He has a limp when he walks, which creates problems with his spine. He already has hyper lordosis and a non-fixed scoliosis. He has balance issues, he falls often. He can't run, he doesn't bend his knees when he walks, which causes knee problems. He can't jump. He gets sick often, with asthmatic bronchitis. He's hyperactive and can't concentrate for more than ten minutes. He can't sit still."

Dr Georgiou takes notes.

He tells me that the diagnosis and research done in France won't tell him much more because none of this information explains the deep underlying reason or cause of Gabrillian's problem. Even if he finds a name for his condition, it won't help him understand how to treat it.

"What does he usually eat? Tell me some dishes that Gabrillian often eats."

"He eats rice, pasta, vegetables. He loves raw carrots, cereal in the morning."

"What kind of cereal?"

"Kellogg's, Chocapic, etc."

"Hmm. I see. What else?"

"Yogurts, apple sauce, chicken and fish. That's with me. At his father's house, he also eats chips, chocolate and drinks fruit juice with meals. I give him fruit juice too, but only between meals, occasionally and in the morning with his breakfast."

"Does he have any food allergies?"

"No. Well, I don't know. How would I know?"

"A good method is to eliminate one type of nutrient at a time. For example, you can try eliminating dairy products and note how he reacts. If you see a clear improvement, you'll have your answer." Dr Georgiou prescribes a dietary plan for Gabrillian.

"No meat! All the livestock in Cyprus is toxic; they are fed with modified soy, I know, I have taken samples myself. Fish is better, but again, not farmed fish because they are also fed with modified soy."

"Gabrillian's father hunts, can I give him game meat?"

"Absolutely not! I have had many cases of hunters poisoned by the lead from their own bullets. Do not give him modified foods, canned foods, ready-made dishes or white flour in any form." I was taking notes in my notebook as fast as I could. These words gave me hope.

"Also, every morning, you will prepare a detoxifying juice for him, based on carrot juice, one-third green juice - you can use coriander, parsley, celery and a beetroot.

You will substitute millet, quinoa, brown or wild rice for pasta and white rice.

Also, no more commercial cereals. You will only give him muesli and oats.

No more milk - you will use rice milk with added calcium, almond milk, or coconut milk."

After some more specific questions about Gabrillian's condition, I understand that the interview appointment has now come to an end.
"Is that all?" I ask.

"For today, yes. I'll give Gabrillian time to adjust before doing these tests. You should come back every two weeks."

At the end of the session, the secretary takes hair samples from Gabrillian from behind his ears and at the occipital level behind his head. Dr Georgiou explains to me that heavy metals exit the body through hair and nails. So, we can identify the presence of circulating heavy metals in the body and the levels of minerals and trace elements from a hair sample.

These are the things I need to action:

- **Define food allergies.**
- **Elimination diet: Exclude one type of food, e.g., dairy products.**
- **Eliminate non-organic meat due to the toxicity of animals fed with modified soy.**
- **No modified foods, no canned foods, no ready-made dishes**
- **No white flour.**
- **No game meat due to the toxicity of lead bullets.**
- **Drink a detoxifying juice every morning: carrot juice, one-third green juice (coriander, parsley, or celery) + one beetroot.**
- **Replace pasta and white rice with millet, quinoa, brown or wild rice.**
- **Replace commercial cereals with muesli or oat flakes.**
- **Replace cow's milk with rice milk, almond milk, or coconut milk with added calcium.**
- **Perform a hair mineral analysis.**

***

December 20, 2016

Two weeks later, we are in Dr Georgiou's office again. I feel a bit embarrassed. Gabrillian has just spilled an entire glass of water on Dr Georgiou's book "Cure the Incurable." Today, my son can't sit still. In the office, he keeps touching everything, wanting to play with the bio resonance machine or the doctor's cards. This is the third time we've come. In a few days, we will go to France for Christmas with family with two days at Disneyland Paris. Gabrillian is very excited.

"Today, we are going to perform a test to detect Gabrillian's food allergies or intolerances," the doctor explains to us. Gabrillian sits on the doctor's table. He loves being taken care of, so he remains very calm.

Dr Georgiou applies a little water to the tip of Gabrillian's index finger and asks me what he eats most often. As I list the different foods, Dr Georgiou is busy, placing and moving small glass tubes containing the molecular identity of the tested element.

He gently presses an electrode on Gabrillian's finger and another in his hand. It reminds me of the phenomenon of electroporation with galvanic current that I learned during my aesthetic BTS (senior technologist's certificate)

(Note: Electroporation or electro permeabilisation is a microbiological technique in which an electric field is applied to cells to increase the permeability of the cell membrane, allowing the introduction of drugs or vitamins into the cell).

I later learned, from browsing a magazine, that this machine was used by NASA following the discovery of the "Quantum Field." Researchers found that matter represents only 0.001% of what we are; the rest is energy - something many ancient traditions have categorised as "chi" or "prana."

This machine explores our energetic relationship with various ingredients, working on the emitted frequency. I would later learn that for an element or remedy to be integrated into Gabrillian's daily life, the relationship between them must emit a frequency of 50. The machine also emits a sound that can be quite discordant if the observed element is not good for Gabrillian. This means that this element will create stress that will later manifest in his physical body.

I also learned that this technique is used in kinesiology. Equal pressure is applied to the outstretched arm of a person and if the person is weakened by a particular thing or thought, the arm falls. Dr Georgiou hands me the analysis sheet for this examination called "Vegatest" and explains to me that Gabrillian has an intolerance of citrus fruits and dairy products. We must avoid cow's milk, goat's milk, as well as all cheeses, all yogurts and Gabrillian can have no butter.

Pulses in general should be avoided, except for lentils. Dr Raj in London will later recommend choosing orange lentils. The worst thing for Gabrillian is that he is not to have sugar in any form. Dr Georgiou explains to me that, for most people, sugar creates inflammation and in Gabrillian's case creates a double inflammation.

"This is the prescription for dietary supplements that Gabrillian must take every day. They are calculated based on Gabrillian's weight, so follow the instructions carefully."

Dr Georgiou lists each supplement and emphasises the quantity, explaining and precisely indicating how to take them and which ones can be mixed with juice and which cannot.

I listen attentively.

He says, "I have also prescribed a series of remedies in case Gabrillian gets sick which you will continue to give him for 7 days after his symptoms cease, to ensure that all microbes disappear. I have also prescribed oregano oil for *you,* in case you get sick."

CHAPTER 5
Radical Changes to Gabrillian's Diet

***

December 2016

I explain the dietary changes we are going to make to Gabrillian in the car and we stop by the supermarket in Pissouri, the village where we live.

"Mom, is this sugar-free? Can I eat it?" Gabrillian asks, picking up various products from the shelves.

And there I am, reading all the labels, checking the contents of products. I'm horrified to see how many products contain sugar or claiming to be "sugar-free" contain something even worse, like aspartame. I remember reading an article explaining how diabetic people were poisoning themselves with these synthetic sweeteners. Sugar with ham? Salt and sugar in ham? What's the point of that?

I also remember that most food chains are owned by the pharmaceutical empire and then suddenly, everything becomes clear.
At first, I get frustrated, but then I realise that ultimately, it's my responsibility to take care of my health and that of my son and if my shopping takes an extra fifteen minutes, I'll do it.

It's morning and I'm getting Gabrillian ready for school before heading to work.

"Gabrillian, come and have breakfast!"

I prepare Gabrillian's juice with a beetroot, two carrots and coriander. Then I add a spoon of Omega fruits, 10 drops of Selenium, 8 drops of HMD (chlorella, cilantro), 0.25 ml of Vitamin D3, a quarter of a spoon of L Glutamine, three-quarters of a spoon of Multi Energy, half a capsule of probiotics (acidophilus + bifidus) and a third of a capsule of Coenzyme Q10 and Vitamin E.

***

A few days later, I hear Gabrillian calling me while I'm cooking and he looks alarmed.

"Mom, Mom, Mom.!" Gabrillian cries.

"What's wrong, Gabrillian?" I ask, concerned.

"Look at my hands!" Gabrillian says, extending them to show me. His fingers are swollen, especially at the tips and I also notice a small red bump next to his nose. I'm anxious, but it's better not to show him because it won't help the situation.

"It's nothing, my little one. We'll call Dr Georgiou tomorrow." I say reassuringly.

The next day, I call Dr Georgiou's office and his secretary puts me through to him.

"Hello, Dr Georgiou, I'm calling because I have a problem. I think my son is reacting to one of the supplements you gave him. Last night, his fingers swelled and red bumps appeared. I think maybe it's the Selenium."

"All right, stop the Selenium for several days and then reintroduce it in small doses. Start with two drops for 3-4 days and if nothing happens, increase the dose by 2 drops again for 4 days and so on, up to a maximum of 8 drops."

Gabrillian goes to his father's house that evening and I'm about to call when suddenly my phone rings.

It's Vassilis.

"Hey, Chori, what are these red bumps on Gabrillian? He's having an allergic reaction to your stuff! I'm warning you, if anything happens to him, it's not going to go well!"

It's in moments like these that I remember and am so grateful for all the techniques of letting go and relaxation that I have learned. I smile, remembering the affirmation that Mira, my hypnotherapist friend, taught me: "Trying to convince others is a considerable waste of energy that could be used more wisely." I take a deep breath, I exhale.

"When I open myself up and allow others the opportunity to express their unique qualities, I discover the treasure of our shared humanity. I release any need to justify myself, seek approval from others, or be right."

I breathe, in and out.

I feel centred, at peace and I ask to speak to Gabrillian's grandmother.

I explain to her that she should stop the Selenium over the weekend and I will reintroduce slowly it into Gabrillian's diet.

Sure enough, after a few days, all the bumps have disappeared.

***

In Summary - Steps to Follow

- Perform a Vega test to determine allergies and intolerances.
- Eliminate sugar in all its forms because it causes inflammation in the body.
- Calculate dietary supplements based on weight.
- Pay attention to how to ingest supplements.
- Beware of "sugar-free" labels: sugar is often replaced with aspartame (carcinogenic).
- Check all labels when grocery shopping.
- Be cautious with Selenium; it can be toxic. Emphasise regenerating the digestive system before introducing Selenium.
- Take natural remedies to treat infections and continue treatment for 7 days after symptoms subside.
- As parents we need to take care of ourselves to have the energy to support our children and not transmit our own issues to our children.

CHAPTER 6
Results of Hair Mineral Analysis

***

January 19, 2017

Today, we received the report of the hair mineral and heavy metals analysis conducted on December 8.

Dr Georgiou hands me the sheet and explains that Gabrillian's minerals and trace elements are at a good level, indicating that he may have absorbed the minerals and vitamins ingested before the examination. However, the levels of arsenic and aluminium are quite high.

"Arsenic may be transferred from the mother to the foetus through the placenta. it is also found in pesticides on vegetables. As for aluminium, I recommend that you throw away all aluminium pots and pans."

Later, I discover that baby rice cereals also contain a lot of arsenic because rice is the cereal that absorbs arsenic from the soil the most. Additionally, Gabrillian had an intolerance to milk when he was younger when the doctor recommended using rice milk. I explain to Dr Georgiou that I was able to reintroduce Selenium in small doses and he recommends that Gabrillian also take a 'cleanse,' a supplement that contains milk thistle, dandelion and burdock root. Dr Georgiou explains that this solution helps detoxify the body and he also adds a Chlorella capsule to remove heavy metals from the organs. Chlorella is one of the most natural supplements used for removing Mercury and other heavy metals. Dr Georgiou explains that the tests conducted only show the circulating heavy metals and with Chlorella, they will detach from the organs and exit through the skin, through respiration, stools and urine.

***

"Chori, I'm taking Gabrillian to the hospital; he has a severe stomach ache!"

I sense seriousness in Vassilis's voice.

"I'm coming right away." I'm worried.

I grab my laptop and some overnight essentials. It's better to be prepared to stay.

When I arrive at the hospital, Vassilis looks serious and Gabrillian, lying on the hospital bed, is clearly in pain.

"My little one!" I say, hugging Gabrillian. He looks very pale and is crying.

"The doctors say it's probably gastroenteritis; they want to keep him under observation tonight." Vassilis says, his tone accusing.

I decide to stay by Gabrillian's bedside. I take out my laptop and ask for the WIFI code. I open my email inbox and find a message from a friend.

"Clémentine, look at this," he writes. The tone is urgent; it must be important. It's about a documentary regarding vaccines, specifically the triple vaccine and its impact on children. The documentary shows that many children are autistic as a direct result of this vaccine.

I watch the documentary, even though I'm very tired. Suddenly, a thought crosses my mind as I see one of the children climbing the stairs and notice the way they walk. Like a duck. Yes, a lot like Gabrillian!

And then I have a flash of inspiration, an 'Aha!' moment.

Gabrillian has been poisoned just like the children in this documentary!

Gabrillian has also had all his vaccines, the DT Polio, the triple vaccine, hepatitis, etc. I must say that at that time, I had done no research. I had simply relied on what the doctor and my parents had recommended. I had no idea about all the effects that vaccines could have.

Later, I would learn from Dr Tatiana, a bio resonance specialist, that Gabrillian's muscular dystrophy may have been caused by the injection of the DT Polio and Tetanus vaccine (see Chapter 18)

Another thought crosses my mind.

If it's toxins that have caused his Muscular Dystrophy, is it possible to eliminate these toxins from his body and heal Gabrillian? I look at Gabrillian, who had finally fallen asleep, his face creased and wet from his discomfort. Even lying in a hospital bed where he was in agony half an hour ago, his healing was, at that moment, a revelation to me—a certainty and a commitment on my part. I will support him on his path to recovery. His "recovery path."

I don’t sleep much that night. I am excited.

In my journal I write the sentence: "Gabrillian is healed."

Key Points

- **Conduct an initial "hair mineral analysis" to determine the number of heavy metals circulating in the body.**
- **Heavy metals accumulate in organs and the brain, emphasising the importance of conducting further "hair mineral" tests after heavy metal detoxification, as they will then circulate in the blood and can be detected.**
- **Arsenic is found in pesticides used on vegetables and grains such as rice.**
- **Aluminium: be cautious and discard all aluminium pots and pans!**
- **The triple vaccine can lead to autistic children.**
- **Heavy metal poisoning can cause motor problems.**

Avoid these Common Mistakes

- **Detoxification that is carried out too fast!**
- **Taking Selenium if digestion and the immune system are weak.**
- **Overlooking the importance of starting the detoxification process at low doses; if there are no bodily reactions, the dose can be gradually increased.**

***

February 9, 2017

"Gabrillian looks a bit pale and you seem exhausted," Dr Georgiou says.

"Yes, Gabrillian had gastroenteritis." I explain, "He went to the hospital. I gave him probiotics, but it didn't prevent him from getting sick again. He constantly has a runny nose and because he is coughing, the doctor tells us to have him inhale Ventolin (salbutamol) three times a day as well as another inhaler with steroids. When it still doesn't improve, the doctor usually prescribes antibiotics and one or two weeks later, he gets sick again."

"How many times has Gabrillian taken antibiotics?" Dr Georgiou asks.

"Since he was a baby." I reply, surprised and a bit embarrassed. I think to myself, there have been so many courses of antibiotics that I can't even remember!

"Ok, approximately. More than 15 times?" Dr Georgiou prompts. I nod and Dr Georgiou's eyes widen.

"That's almost a crime!" he exclaims.

He regains his composure and tells me that we will put Gabrillian on a program to boost his immune system because every time Gabrillian comes into contact with a germ, he catches it and that's not normal.

He prescribes two supplements—Immunfor and Epicor—for three months. It's a mixture of different mushrooms such as Reishi and Neem.

He also recommends that Gabrillian drink ginger and elderberry flower infusions.

While the doctor explains this, to keep him quiet, I give Gabrillian my mobile phone to watch cartoons.

"Does he always hold the screen so close to his face?" Dr Georgiou asks. "Excuse me, but whenever I see children of his age hypnotised by mobile phone screens or iPads, it makes my hair stand on end. Electromagnetic waves are not good for adults; they disrupt the hormonal system, but for a child Gabrillian's age, the waves penetrate up to a quarter of the brain. For a baby, it's half of the brain."

Suddenly a light dawns and I realise that it's not surprising that Gabrillian sleeps so poorly after playing on or watching my phone. I feel ashamed. But if I hadn't given him the cartoons, we wouldn't have been able to have a consultation without constant interruptions. But I promise myself to limit Gabrillian's use of the phone as much as possible.

"Have you noticed any differences or improvements in Gabrillian's condition?" Dr Georgiou asks.

"Yes, Gabrillian seems more confident in himself and his legs are stronger now!" I reply. "He tries to go down the stairs without holding onto the wall! He challenges himself to improve. It seems like he has more confidence in himself. Also, I've noticed that he's a bit calmer and less aggressive at home."

"How would you evaluate Gabrillian's progress?" Dr Georgiou asks.
The image of Gabrillian yesterday on the stairs comes to my mind. Gabrillian stands at the top of the stairs without handrails in the house.

"Look at me, Mom!" Gabrillian exclaims excitedly, coming down the stairs, standing, holding onto the wall a little. And to think that a few months ago, he would come down the stairs on his bottom and tear all his pants!

"I would say about a 25% improvement," I reply with a smile. "That's fantastic, congratulations!" Dr Georgiou exclaims. He is delighted with Gabrillian's progress and so am I!

***

In Summary Key Takeaways from this Chapter

- Define food allergies, intolerances and reduce heavy metals.
- Implement an exclusion diet.
- Certain foods can trigger skin reactions, bowel issues, pain, fatigue, headaches, etc. To detect these sensitivities, Dr Georgiou recommended starting with an exclusion diet. It involves:

- Excluding one category of foods (dairy products, gluten, etc.) at a time for a minimum of one week to a month.
- Monitoring clinical improvement: maintain a daily journal with meal compositions, bodily reactions, stool condition.
- Reintroduce that food; this is called a provocation test, to assess whether the food intolerance exists based on the reaction (urgency, hives, stomach pain, hyperactivity, etc.).
- If this food triggers an allergic reaction, it is recommended that you:
- Eliminate that ingredient for at least 6 months and reintroduce it once a week into the diet as a treat.
- Take refreshing herbs regularly to support the gastrointestinal canal membranes, such as Milk Thistle or Gentian.
- Take homeopathic remedies.
- Take Bach Flower Remedies to keep the body free from tension.

To soothe allergies, I found the following helpful:

- Mangosteen juice: it's a very potent antioxidant that can help shield the body from free radical stress. It's an excellent anti-inflammatory to counteract inflammation caused by allergens, especially since, in the beginning, due to the damage to the intestinal mucosa, the person or child is fundamentally allergic to almost everything. I found it to be excellent support for staying healthy during the transition phase.

- Frankincense, 2 drops under the tongue morning and evening, works wonders for soothing food allergies and supporting the immune system.

Avoid common allergens:

- Sugar
- Lactose: dairy products in general.

Dr Mathieu, hepatogastroenterologist, CHU Grenoble, France: "There are 4.5 billion people on Earth who do not digest dairy products."

Children are often more allergic to lactose than adults. It is usually a form of intolerance that creates an over-fermentation of intestinal flora.

To treat this intolerance:

- Exclude all lactose-containing products for a period of 6 months
- Reintroduce a maximum of 12 grams of lactose per day, for example a Greek yogurt or some cottage cheese-style cheese.
- Add supplements such as enzymes or even herbal supplements to support intestinal mucosa during absorption (e.g., Aloe Vera, mangosteen).
- Favour fermented and goat dairy products once the person or child is ready for this stage.

- When dairy is cultured for at least 24 hours, almost all of the lactose is pre-digested, making it easy to digest for the sensitive individual.

Examples of cultured dairy:

- Ghee
- Cultured butter
- Sour cream or Cultured Cream
- Yogurt
- Kefir

- Use alternatives such as coconut milk or almond milk.
- Avoid Gluten, a protein found in wheat, barley and rye grains and exclusively found in the seed of the plant, which is ground to be used as flour. You'll find it in:

- Barley
- Rye
- Wheat
- Bread
- Commercial cereals, muesli, oats
- Pasta

Alternatives to use:

- Buckwheat. It's not wheat; it's not even a true grain. It should also be labelled gluten-free because it can sometimes be cross-contaminated.
- Gluten-free oats. Quinoa and Millet are reasonably good options too.

- FODMAPs – fermentable oligosaccharides (fructans, galacto- oligosaccharides), disaccharides (lactose), monosaccharides (fructose) and polyols (sorbitol, mannitol, xylitol, maltitol): These are found in foods like garlic, onions, peas, lentils, peaches, melons, pomegranates, grapes, sausages, honey, milk, apples, pears, asparagus, beets, cabbage, beans, coffee, parsley, leeks.

Sensitivity can vary from person to person. For example, my son is sensitive to beans, but he can eat red lentils.

All dairy products are rich in FODMAPs and rye and barley are rich in fructans and galactans.

- Do a Vega test.
- Conduct a hair mineral analysis.

Mistakes to Avoid :

- Not checking with the bio-resonance machine for compatibility of remedies with the person being treated. A certain brand of supplements can have different components that may be incompatible with the individual and create unnecessary inflammations in the body that are easy to avoid.
- Skipping steps and giving heavy metal detoxifiers or chelators too quickly.
- Being too aggressive and not gradual enough!

A Prescription to Boost the Immune System

Immunfor: neem, reish, ginger infusion

***

CHAPTER 7

Visit to Dr Raj Bhachu in London

***

February 14, 2017

We took the plane early this morning. We arrived in London around 11 a.m.

"Gabrillian, come here!" Every time I turn my head, he has sneaked off somewhere! I keep calling him back to me.

I look at the stroller. We ended up using it to carry the luggage since Gabrillian doesn't seem interested in sitting in it. Finally, he gets tired and wants to sit.

We wait in line to get a ticket for the subway. I can see that Gabrillian is already getting impatient. Krasimir is getting involved now and my son sits down.

I wonder how Gabrillian can be both so restless and easily fatigued to the point that sometimes even his eyes droop with tiredness. He has the energy to crawl under and open all the airport barriers, but not to walk more than 100 meters or chew a beef steak!

We finally arrive in Northwood Hills, not without getting lost once or twice.

Later we satisfy our hunger at a small restaurant. Gabrillian eats two fried eggs, probably fried in sunflower oil and unusually, some fries.

Gabrillian has no idea that this will be the last time he eats fries.

On the ground floor is the main reception for the various offices on the upper floors and after introducing ourselves, Bella, Dr Raj's secretary, comes to fetch us.

The reception is welcoming and Gabrillian immediately looks comfortable.

"So, tell me, how can I help you? What is concerning you about Gabrillian's condition?" Dr Raj asks.

I explain to him that the tests are inconclusive and we still don't have a definitive diagnosis.

Dr Raj interrupts me and asks me to stick to the symptoms. I describe Gabrillian's various symptoms: his gait, balance and coordination issues, atrophies in both quadriceps, his hyperactivity and his fatigue.

Dr Raj also asks for medical history, from my side and Gabrillian's father's side.

"And you? Do you have any health problems?" Dr Raj asks. "On my side, I have a cousin with myasthenia gravis (which I now know comes from ancient Greek and Latin and means 'serious muscle weakness') and a great-uncle with multiple sclerosis. My mother died when I was young, of breast cancer. My immune system is rather weak because I often have different infections."

"Is that all? And the father?" Dr Raj asks, clearly surprised.

"Vassilis has a brother with quite serious rheumatism. He has to take daily injections for the pain. As for Vassilis, he had panic attacks while I was pregnant. He also constantly suffers from acid reflux and irritable bowel syndrome."

Dr Raj takes notes.

He asks Gabrillian to remove his socks.

Dr Raj laughs upon seeing that Gabrillian is also wearing tights under his pants.

"You come from a warm place, right? It's very cold here for you."
I explain to Dr Raj that Gabrillian always has cold feet. He has trouble warming up and at night, he always asks for an extra blanket. And when I check on him before going to bed, I notice that he's now extremely warm although he hasn't uncovered himself and he's always covered in sweat.

It's as if he doesn't have the ability to feel his body temperature.
Dr Raj begins evaluating Gabrillian's condition.

He also uses a bio resonance machine, but his technique is completely different from Dr Georgiou's.

He starts with Gabrillian's hands.

Every time he evaluates a finger with the machine, he applies a little water to the fingertips or sometimes even to the finger joints, to increase conductivity.

He explains to me that on this or that finger, he can detect an imbalance related to an organ, gland, or system.

Next he works with Gabrillian's feet and toes, which also, he tells me, correspond to other organs.

I listen and watch, fascinated, as he inputs data about the health of each of Gabrillian's organs.

Gabrillian allows it and seems interested in Dr Raj's work. Dr Raj tells me that Gabrillian has thyroid problems and that most of his organs and glands are imbalanced.

"But don't worry, we'll address that," he reassures me.

After the evaluation, he places the dietary supplements recommended by Dr Georgiou for my son on the machine while Gabrillian holds an electrode in his hand.

Dr Raj then places the other electrode, shaped like a pen, on Gabrillian's left-hand fingers to evaluate their compatibility with his remedies.

He checks them one by one and tells me that only two supplements are good for Gabrillian - a mother tincture based on Neem to boost his immune system and various mushrooms. The Bach Flower Remedy prepared by Dr Georgiou also turns out to be a very good remedy for my son.

I would later learn the reasons behind why Gabrillian made progress with some supplements and experienced skin reactions and intestinal problems with others.

I would also discover later that when a person has a leaky gut, they become intolerant to almost everything. Gabrillian may have absorbed some nutrients initially, but his body later had an allergic reaction to them.

Also, Selenium is a heavy metal and can turn into poison for the body if the person is deficient in essential minerals.

Dr Raj opens another box containing multiple small samples, which he places on the machine in place of the supplements. "Isn't it strange that vaccines didn't cause Gabrillian's problems? Did you or your husband ever use hard drugs in the past?" "No, I have not and I'm sure that for Vassilis, the answer is also no."
"Yeah, you don't look like the type!" Dr Raj replies, smiling.

Dr Raj now places various herbal and homeopathic remedies in a metal bowl on the machine, intended to test my son's energy compatibility with these supplements. I watch him remove and exchange different supplements and test again and again with different fingers corresponding to different organs, until finally, he finds the perfect combination for Gabrillian's immune, respiratory, cardiac, endocrine and all corresponding organs and glands.
Finally, he is satisfied with his findings.

"My secretary will explain to you how to use these herbal remedies and we will also provide you with a list of foods that Gabrillian can eat. It's going to be tough, very tough, but you must do it! From now on, you'll have to eliminate all gluten from his diet! No more dairy products and no more sugar!"

Initially, I wondered, why gluten? Dr Georgiou hadn't mentioned that Gabrillian was gluten intolerant. I would later learn that dairy products and gluten prevent nutrient absorption by creating a kind of 'glue' in the intestinal mucosa.

In my son's case, it made perfect sense to avoid such foods so as not to exacerbate the problem of malnutrition.

"You'll make him toast with rice cakes and almond butter; it's delicious! For breakfast, soft-boiled eggs with avocado slices. The key is how you prepare it."

"What can I give him instead of gluten?" I asked, concerned. "You'll give him white basmati rice (not brown rice; it's hard to digest), quinoa (but not too much as it can inflame the digestive tract), red lentils (orange colour). Later on, you can also make your own bread with pea flour."

"Will Gabrillian ever be able to eat dairy products?"

"Afterward, he'll be able to have cottage cheese on his toast. For now, we'll focus on a protein-rich diet with good fats and low carbohydrates. Animal proteins help build muscles and maintain high energy levels without causing insulin spikes. For animal proteins, you'll give him poultry, a bit of beef, rabbit, non-farmed fish and free-range chicken eggs. The key for meat is the source; prioritise organic and lean meats."

Recipe for Dr Raj's Chicken Bone Broth

Ingredients

1 whole organic free-range chicken or 1 kg of bony chicken parts, such as necks, backs, breastbones and wings

Gizzards (optional)
2-4 chicken feet (optional)
4 litres of filtered cold water
2 tablespoons of apple cider vinegar
1 large onion, roughly chopped
3 celery stalks, roughly chopped
2 carrots, peeled and roughly chopped
1 bunch of parsley

Preparation

If you are using a whole chicken, cut off the wings, remove the neck, fat glands and gizzards from the cavity.

Cut the chicken pieces into several parts.

Place the chicken or chicken pieces in a large stainless-steel pot with water, vinegar and all the vegetables except for the parsley. Let it sit for 30 minutes.

Bring to a boil and skim off the scum that rises to the surface. Reduce the heat, cover and simmer for 6-8 hours.

The longer you cook the broth, the richer and more flavourful it will be.

About 10 minutes before you finish the broth, add the parsley. This will add extra mineral ions to the broth.

Remove the whole chicken or chicken pieces with a slotted spoon.
If you're using a whole chicken, let it cool and remove the chicken meat from the carcass and set it aside for other uses such as chicken salads.

Strain the broth into a large bowl and let it sit until the fat rises to the surface and congeals.

Remove this fat and store the broth in covered containers in your refrigerator or freezer.

***

A few weeks later, I speak with Dr Raj on Skype.

"Hello, Clémentine, how are you? How is Gabrillian doing?"
"Thank you, I'm fine. Gabrillian is doing well generally, but he still has diarrhoea and he's not gaining weight."

"It will pass, you'll see. Later on, his muscles will grow as well. But wait, I'm going to get a colleague to show you a technique that you can use with Gabrillian to regulate this problem."

Dr Raj directs the camera towards the back of his colleague, sitting on a stool. He explains to me:

"You will measure, about two fingers, thumb and index, below the hairline on the neck; you will use Gabrillian's finger measurements and press six times with the edges of both hands, like this, then another six times below and again six times."
Dr Raj shows me how to stimulate acupuncture points by applying pressure to the edges of hands and I recognise the bladder meridian. This stimulation helps regulate the excess energy in the bladder meridian and thus regulates the lack of energy in the kidney meridian, which is the root cause of digestion and absorption issues.

"Can I use honey or agave syrup for Gabrillian?" I asked Dr Raj.

"No, agave syrup is not good for him. I prefer cinnamon or Yemeni honey. Look it up online and you'll see the properties of this 'superfood.'"

"Gabrillian's father always gives him sugar and yogurt." I say, nervously.
"Give me his phone; I'm going to call him right now and explain how important this is!" Dr Raj is very serious.

***

May 2017. Second appointment in London.

Five months pregnant, with a backpack on my shoulders filled with our clothes for the next day, I push an empty stroller. I watch Gabrillian slip between the flimsy barriers separating the lines of airport passengers. It's as if Gabrillian had a sixth sense and could feel the frustration, impatience and annoyance of the people waiting in line. Maybe he could even sense their own mischievous desire to undo all these barriers and break free from the rules!

Then, suddenly, he couldn't wait anymore. He looks at me smiling from ear to ear and starts undoing the barriers! Not only does he not listen, but he also taunts me!

How do I stop him? He's already slipped into the first rows! "Whose child is this?" demands the customs officer.

Red with shame, I say "he's my son."

"Please come get him!" the British agent tells me officiously. I squeeze past the people in the queue, who look at me angrily. I grab Gabrillian and I promise him that he'll hear from me and that he'll be without his iPad for a while.

He grumbles and cries a little, but it doesn't last.

We finally arrive at a beautiful Edwardian-style house on Murray Street in Northwood Hills. I had found this bed and breakfast on Airbnb.
Gabrillian is now so tired from all his escapades at the airport that he hasn't moved from his stroller, except in the underground where he couldn't help but dance between the doors. I thought my heart was going to stop, but in the end, we survived. "Finally, I'll be able to rest." I said to myself.

We ring the doorbell and another little boy comes to greet us with his parents. We introduce ourselves. At that moment, I notice that Gabrillian has disappeared into the host's kitchen and is asking the hostess for food. Embarrassed, I grab Gabrillian by the hand and explain that we're about to go out to eat. At that moment, he sees the piano.

"No, Gabrillian, don't touch that!" I call out helplessly. He's already pounding the piano keys.

I finally manage to detach him from the piano and guide him to our room.

"Just play here for a minute; I'm going to the bathroom." I say. I have not even got the bathroom door shut before I hear him playing the piano again. I'm about to go to him when I hear the lady of the house telling Gabrillian not to play on this piano, explaining that it has been in their family for a very long time and that it's very old. She offers him maracas instead. He doesn't seem particularly excited.

We go out for dinner. I decide to try our luck in the small town of Northwood. I think that for once, I can let him eat what he wants. After all, Dr Raj even told us not to bring his remedies with us. Gabrillian orders spaghetti bolognese - he loves that - and also a small dessert.

He is already crawling under the table. Gabrillian starts running all over the restaurant hiding under the other tables. Embarrassed, I quickly finish my plate, pay the bill and we disappear into the street.

"Gaby, stay in your stroller! If you keep doing this, you'll go by yourself all the way home! I'll leave you all alone!" I say, irritated. He doesn't hear me. He's in his own world and fast becoming uncontrollable. He just can't stay in one place.

Finally, we arrive at the Edwardian house and all I want is to take a long shower and sleep. But Gabrillian has decided otherwise. He wants to go outside to play with the little boy he saw when we arrived. Finally, I calm him down by offering him my iPad so that I can have some peace while I take a shower.

When I come back into the room, Gabrillian has calmed down. I change him and he finally falls asleep. Lying next to my little boy, the night before our appointment with Dr Raj, a thousand thoughts flood into my mind from all directions. I finally manage to fall asleep.

***

The next morning, our host brings us breakfast at 7 a.m. as agreed. It's a wonderful, varied breakfast with Weetabix, fruits, scones, milk and tea. I wonder how to ask them, after all their efforts, if they could just make us two fried eggs. I swallow hard and think that to do without for once, won't hurt him. What a mistake!

Our host drops us off in front of Dr Raj's office as planned and I thank her for her hospitality and help.

I spot Dr Raj with his students, discussing his method. I later learned that Dr Raj teaches his technique. He explained to me that it can take more than a year to train students. Gabrillian is excited in the elevator. He absolutely wants to talk to Dr Raj. His English is not very good at this point, so he keeps asking me.

"Mom, Mom, tell Dr Raj I ate sweet things!"

Gabrillian takes out his little book in which his grandmother and I have described all of Gabrillian's meals and also his digestive and other reactions, if there were any.

Dr Raj asks me to read a few pages to get an idea of what Gabrillian eats.

"Friday, June 9th, for breakfast, he had two soft-boiled eggs and half an avocado."

"Very good."

"For a snack, an apple, a rice cake with peanut butter."

"Prefer almond butter."

"His grandmother also gives him a lot of rabbit and chicken. He generally eats a lot of salmon and sea bream."

"That's good."

"Mom, Mom." Gabrillian insists, tugging at my arm.

"We also give him a lot of sweet potatoes to replace regular potatoes. His grandmother also gives him agave syrup instead of honey."
"Mom, Mom, tell Dr Raj that." Gabrillian interrupts me.

"That's not good; it's better to use cinnamon or Yemeni honey," Dr Raj reminds me.

I observe Dr Raj checking all the organs and glands with the bio resonance machine. He applies a little water to Gabrillian's fingertips. The machine makes a rather harmonious sound. I am surprised and ask Dr Raj if his condition has improved. "Look at the colours!" Dr Raj exclaims, showing me the computer screen where the main organs, glands and endocrine systems are classified one by one.

The dominant colour is neutral. Only two lines are still red. "Gabrillian is much better. All the indices are close to 50, which is normal. Only the gallbladder and spleen are still imbalanced."

"How is his personal life now?"

I remember that the first time Dr Raj was surprised to see this imbalance in his personal life.

"It's still not good."

"I'll give you something for that."

"Have you noticed any changes in Gabrillian since your last visit?"

I nodded, "I would say he's less sick; his immune system seems to have improved. He seems to digest better, has less diarrhoea and is generally calmer. However, he has only gained 500 grams in weight since the last time I saw you."

"You'll see, Clémentine, after this, his muscles will grow. For now, his digestive system needs to be perfect and then we'll work on the muscles."

I remember that when Gabrillian took Co-Enzyme Q10, Selenium and vitamin D, he was stronger in his legs.

Dr Raj prescribes other supplements for my son and a new remedy called MTB-Tox. I read the following description online: MTB-Tox is a unique homeopathic formula designed to address geopathic stress and the "imponderables" and provide the resonances needed for the life force to bring about healing and resolution.

I look at Gabrillian. He clearly can't take it anymore; he jumps around, over excited.

"What did Gabrillian eat last night and this morning?" Dr Raj asks me, looking a little concerned, as he watches him.

I explain to Dr Raj about the spaghetti from yesterday and the Weetabix this morning.

"Oh, that's why!" he says. "That explains everything!"

"Can the effects work so quickly and with only two servings?" I ask in astonishment.

"Of course!" Dr Raj assures me.

"At school, he still eats cookies; the teacher complains that she barely turns her back and he has another child's snack. Sometimes he even takes them from their bags and hides to eat them."
"You can't control that; he always wants to eat those things. But at home, you can set your own rules and be strict."

"What exactly happens to him when he eats sweet things or gluten?"
"It gives him a slap in the brain and he doesn't understand what's happening to him."

And just like that, it all became clear. Yes, that was why every time he eats those things, he became hysterical, uncontrollable. It's as if he feels embarrassed, uncomfortable and doesn't know how to express it. Even when he had back pain due to his poor posture and gait, he didn't know how to say it and if I massaged his back, he said it tickled and wriggled all over the place. I decide I will have to be stricter at home.

Suddenly, Gabrillian grabs a hard cushion and hits me right on the nose. Tears well up in my eyes. I already have allergies, a swollen nose and red eyes, but this was adding insult to injury! I hear Dr Raj reprimanding Gabrillian.

"Don't do that; this is the person who takes care of you," he explains to Gabrillian.

"Are you okay, Clémentine?"

I'm so tired and with the throbbing pain and humiliation, I start crying. Gabrillian looks at me, not knowing exactly what to do, but he knows he's made a mistake.

Later, he will apologise for his actions.

I also learned later that children like Gabrillian, with attention deficit problems, often lack empathy as well. Often they hit or even bite the people they love the most, or who are closest to them. It's a matter of biochemistry, neuron receptors they are almost compelled even if they don't want to, the urge is stronger than they are. It comes under the heading of 'behavioural disorders.' When I ask Dr Raj if he has other cases like Gabrillian's, he assures me that he has seen much worse.

We decide to focus our attention on Gabrillian's gastric problems in the coming weeks, especially repairing his leaky gut syndrome. We are about to leave Dr Raj's office. Bella, the secretary, is preparing the homeopathic remedies for Gabrillian. She also offers us a glass of a fantastic Fiji mineral water, which Dr Raj also recommends using. Fiji water is extracted from an artesian aquifer in the Fiji Islands and is rich in silicon, magnesium and calcium, giving it a very mild taste. Dr Raj also provides me with a list of mineral waters that he recommends, such as Volvic water. I notice the other secretary working in a laboratory at the back of the office, presumably producing more remedies. I see her holding a bottle of vodka, the alcohol necessary for creating this type of remedy. You have to let the plants or roots macerate for weeks. I learned that when I studied herbal medicine. Bella explains how to make up the remedies.

"You'll mix 10 drops each of mother tincture in 700 ml of water."

"Can I split it half-and-half and give him this mixture once in the morning and once in the evening?" I ask, "because when he goes to school, I can't control how much water he drinks and he might exchange his bottle with another child."

"I understand. Let me ask Dr Raj about that."

She comes back and tells me that there's no problem with splitting the remedy into two large glasses of water.

"I can also confirm that you can use boiling water to evaporate the alcohol in the remedies."

We leave Dr Raj's office and prepare to take 4 subways, 2 hours of bus rides, hours of waiting at the airport and finally, a 5-hour flight back to Cyprus.

It's going to be a long day!

***

Later, at the airport

"Madam, you'll have to take everything out for me." The customs officer at Gatwick Airport is looking suspiciously at the amount of medication I have in my case.

"I have my son's doctor's prescription," I stammer. He looks at it. "I see, yes, that's OK," he says.

I have unpacked all my bags to get all the bottles of homeopathic remedies out and in the meantime, Gabrillian has already escaped and is climbing on all the tables provided for the bags to be put on to be examined.

"Madam, is that your son?" the officer is beginning to get impatient.

I nod my head, embarrassed.

"Can you please tell him to come down?" the customs officer is now openly irritated.

"Gabrillian! Gabrillian! Get down!" I shout.

But Gabrillian, under the influence of gluten and sugar, was already lost in his own world and could no longer hear anything I said. He had already lost all visual contact with me and anyone trying to communicate with him.

***

On the plane, Gabrillian found it difficult to sit still, he slipped out under his seat and walked in the plane aisle, trying to find someone to play with. In the seats in front of us, two little girls had fits of the giggles every two minutes especially when Gabrillian was being goofy. When they turned away, Gabrillian, in an effort to regain their attention, pulled on one of the little girl's pigtails.

“Daddy daddy” she wailed and her father turned to console her.
“What's the matter, sweetheart?”
“That little boy behind me pulled my hair!” She pointed an accusatory finger at Gabrillian.
I apologise hastily.

“Gabrillian, I say gently, “It’s not nice to pull the little girl's hair, because it hurts her.”
The little girl is peeping at us between the seats and now turns around, deliberately placing her pigtail in the gap between the seats, where Gabrillian can reach it. Before I could stop him Gabrillian has reached for the dangling hair, giving it a tug.

Her father, alerted by a new exaggerated wail from his daughter, presses the button for the flight attendant and asks that they be allowed to change seats because the boy behind was bothering his daughter.

I felt a mixture of anger and embarrassment, the father had totally overreacted to his daughter's mischievous behaviour, she actually reminded me of my sister and countless similar incidents that had coloured our childhood. The little girl and Gabrillian would, if left to themselves, have tired of that game fairly quickly and found something else to amuse themselves with. The father's escalation of the issue removed that possibility and left all of us feeling tense and unhappy.
In Larnaca airport, as we disembarked and joined the queue for immigration, Gabrillian gave me the slip again as he ducked under the ropes of the lanes. I had to chase him through rows of disgruntled passengers. I could see from their faces that they blamed me for not being able to control my son. I caught up with him beside the man who had been seated in front of us on the plane, with his daughters. His disdain was obvious as he said.
“I see that once again, you and your child are causing problems.”

I felt a helpless rage threaten to make me explode. Here I was, 5 months pregnant travelling with my son for two days and nobody could show us even the slightest sympathy or compassion. Of course, they didn't know what I was dealing with, but even the most basic human kindness or even a smile would have felt like a million dollars to me at that moment. My backpack was digging into my shoulders and I was manhandling Gabrillian’s stroller that

he only used when he was very tired. None of this put me in a position to be fast enough to catch up with my son! As the man and his daughters stared at me, I simply felt exhausted, frustrated and angry and all I could manage in return was,
"What's your problem?"

Finally, we made it to the exit where Vassilis was waiting to pick us up. I had left my car at his parent's house. He had made a big deal about taking us to the airport, probably because he felt guilty for not coming with us to speak to Doctor Raj, Gabrillian's doctor. That had been a recurring theme with Vasilis. It was as though he was in denial and if he didn't come to appointments, he wouldn't have to confront the fact that there was something wrong with Gabrillian that could not be fixed with a pill.

As we drove away from the airport, I told Vasilis that we were going to have to make some changes in Gabrillian's diet. Vasilis sighed deeply.

"You know, I really don't believe in all of this."
That was the last straw.
"Are you kidding me?" I raged "I've been dragging Gabrillian around for the last two days, I'm exhausted and he can't sit still and we are being insulted by other people because of his behaviour and all you can say is you don't believe in all this!" I was boiling over now. "You didn't have to do anything to help us, did you? You chose to go down this route. Perhaps now you would prefer to see Gabrillian in a wheelchair gradually deteriorating, would that suit you better?"
Now Vasilis turned to me and I could smell alcohol on his breath.
"Shut up! I'm warning you, Clementine, you're really pushing me now!"

We arrived at his parent's house and I jumped out of the car and with shaking hands, started my own car and drove away. A little way down the road I stopped the car and rested my head on my arms over the steering wheel. The floodgates opened and I wept a mixture of tears of sorrow and anger, love and frustration. Later that evening Vasilis sent me a message of apology.

At home, I went to bed, the events of the day replaying in my head on a loop. Suddenly I had a revelation. Everything that happened, every disapproving look or insult directed at me, I had taken personally, making myself a victim and giving all those that I had come up against, a stick to beat me with.

I got out of bed and went to the bathroom and looked at myself in the mirror. Was I ready to shake free of my victim status? In my mind, I replayed the scene in Dr Raj's office when Gabrillian had hit me with a cushion. As that scene replayed in my mind I was suddenly transported back to my teenage years when I had wanted to hide away, ashamed and deeply self-conscious about the acne that covered my cheeks.

Looking at myself in another mirror all those years ago, each day I'd hated myself a little bit more.

"Look at yourself, you're so ugly you don't even deserve to exist!" I would hiss at my reflection. At those times, the urge to hurt myself or even end my tortured existence was almost overwhelming.

No one else seemed to realise what anguish I was in. My sister would look at me and say accusingly.

"You're not the only one with pimples you know, there are lots of people with more pimples than you, don't make such a fuss!"

In my misery, I would snap back.

"Yes and then there are some people like you who have no pimples at all! It's just so unfair, why me?"

Another image now played in my mind. I was in a physical education class at school playing handball. I dreaded any moment that I would get the ball because I hated having attention drawn to me. Without warning, I was hit in the face with the ball with such force that it took my breath away. My nose was hurting badly and I could feel tears welling up in my eyes. The boy who had thrown the ball was very quick to apologise but all I could hear was the deafening roar of my shame and anger, ringing in my ears. My mouth opened in a torrent of abuse, hurled at the boy, as my anger spewed out.

Now I heard Doctor Raj's voice asking, "What can I do for you, Clementine?" It was an echo of the scene in his office that morning. I found myself staring into the mirror, struggling to make the connection between the scenes that my brain was projecting into my consciousness. What was the message? Had I somehow determined the outcome of these encounters myself, by having a victim mentality? Was this a message that if I didn't want to be treated like a victim I would have to lose the victim mentality? The uncertainty, the self-loathing and feeling ashamed - they were all determining how things turned out for me and how others perceived me. It was time to let them go.

I stood up tall and looked myself straight in the eye in the mirror, my image distorted by the tears that overflowed my eyes. My throat felt tight and sore but I spoke these words out loud.

"I forgive myself for judging myself as being unworthy of the love or receiving attention and for falling short of my own expectations. I forgive my parents for not always knowing how to show me my value or how to give me the attention I needed." I finished my promise to myself by saying.
"Clementine, I love you anyway and in every way."

As tears continued to flow down my cheeks I smiled at myself. Bizarrely the story of Narcissus who stared at his reflection too long came to mind. I smiled again. It turns out that looking at yourself without a filter and with brutal honesty takes courage!

Now, I felt lighter, I could almost feel the victim mentality that had been part of me for so long, drifting away. The 'victim'

Clementine may not have gone far and I have no doubt she will return, but when she does reappear, I will be ready for her!

Turning off the bathroom light I returned to bed and a deep, peaceful, replenishing sleep.

CHAPTER 8
Meeting Todd Harrison

***

March 2017

Mark had sent me an email. It contained various internet links to videos that he asked me to watch. I clicked on the link and found myself on the "Beat Muscular Dystrophy" website with multiple videos of a young man named Todd Harrison. He was in his twenties and had been diagnosed with Becker muscular dystrophy when he was young.

I watched a video where Todd Harrison presented a range of supplements:
"I am currently on a complete dietary supplement program that includes the following Youngevity products: 'Beyond Tangy Tangerine,' 'OsteoFx,' 'EFA Plus,' 'Gluco gel capsules,' 'Ultimate Selenium,' 'HGH Youth Complex,' and 'Z Radical,' which you can see behind me."

I opened another video showing Todd's improvements in physical performance. He could go down the stairs faster, his gait had improved, his feet didn't turn outward as much and what struck me the most was the endurance he had! He was doing sit-ups, push-ups. It was impressive! I couldn't believe it!

I also learned about Todd's progress after using Dr Donald Rhodes' "Vecttor" machine in Houston for six months, a machine that helps deliver nutrients to cells through electroporation. He could jump skilfully and could easily lift a chair! Wow! Todd Harrison had been diagnosed with Becker muscular dystrophy at the age of 3. In his family, two of his uncles had already died from this condition.

However, Todd showed determination and confidence in seeking solutions. He was determined not to end up in a wheelchair. So, he began to browse through hundreds of magazines, newspapers and any books he could find on this subject until one day, he came across an article explaining how to treat muscular dystrophy in sheep. His discoveries didn't stop there and shortly after, he met the author of that article, naturopathic doctor Joel Wallach, who would later become his mentor.

Joel Wallach is the founder of the Youngevity company. I would later learn that he started as a veterinarian after earning his degree from the agricultural school. He then worked in Africa and the United States, where he was responsible for conducting autopsies to find the causes of deaths in certain animals sensitive to pollution. There, he made a very important discovery: the deaths of these animals were actually caused by nutritional deficiencies! Later, he became a naturopath to transfer the benefits of his work to the human race.

On the "Beat MD" website, on the page titled "The Conceptual Revolution of Muscular Dystrophy," I discovered the following statements:

"Muscular dystrophy or muscle atrophy simply means 'malnutrition or lack of nutrition to muscles!'"

"When you add Selenium to the diet, the symptoms of muscular dystrophy disappear!"

"Not all regions of the world have the same proportion of Selenium in their soils, which explains why some regions like

Keshan in China—where there is no Selenium in the soil—are high-risk areas and the number of people suffering from Muscular Dystrophy is much higher."

"A dietary deficiency in Selenium can cause DNA mutation!"

"A deficiency of micronutrients can lead to DNA degradation, such as chromosome breaks in human cell cultures or in vitro!"

"Prednisone, a drug commonly used in the treatment of Muscular Dystrophy, increases Selenium deficiency."

"Vitamin E is an essential cofactor for Selenium to function properly."

"In 1983, a study was conducted by Dr Gustav Orndahl on five patients suffering from Muscular Dystrophy. They were given a high dose of Selenium and Vitamin E. The results were surprising. All five patients improved in different ways; one increased grip strength and the others gait improved, with better alignment."

Wow! I was amazed. But I was beginning to realise that the solution was becoming more and more evident—that is, to try to provide Gabrillian's cells with the maximum and best quality of nutrition, especially his muscle cells! It just might help.

I looked at Gabrillian lying in his hospital bed. Despite not having slept a wink all night, when the first rays of sunshine filtered through the window curtains, I was initially blinded, but then I finally saw the end of the tunnel. The end of this long nightmare. At the other end, I could finally see a glimmer of hope.

I suddenly felt very light and a newfound enthusiasm revived my heart.

I now knew that Gabrillian could be cured. I grabbed my pen and with a determined smile, I wrote again in my journal: "Gabrillian is cured!"

***

A few days later, I found a "Beat Muscular Dystrophy" page on Facebook and decided to send a message to Todd Harrison. To my surprise, he responded fairly quickly and we started chatting regularly.

I described the dietary regimen and the dietary supplements was I using to him. I also sent him videos showing examples of Gabrillian's physical performance. A video showing how he walks, how he runs—or rather, walks quickly—how he can't jump. He explained to me that based on his experience with various cases of muscular dystrophy, it seemed to be a case of muscular dystrophy myopathy.

After sending him photos of the various supplements recommended by the naturopath, he explained that he was interested in the liquid form of the Omega solution. He explained that oils need to be encapsulated to avoid contact with air, which would lead to rancidity and render the oils ineffective.

He later told me that this was the reason Gabrillian had a skin reaction. Selenium is a heavy metal that can be toxic if not given in the proper dose and not in a neutral form. He said that once Todd and the families found the right dosage of Selenium, the results were impressive!

Todd sent me a video of a 4-year-old child who couldn't walk. He held onto his mother's arm, had no balance and his head was tilted completely backward. This was followed by another video of the same boy, after 3 and a half months on the correct dosage of Selenium and Youngevity supplements. Now I saw a child who could walk without assistance. It was very encouraging!

Todd also studied Gabrillian's multivitamin complex and explained the theory to me, that the body needs 90 essential nutrients to function properly.

Todd gave me the example of baking a cake: "It's like making a cake; you can't just use flour; you need other ingredients. And it's the same with the right dosage."

"Do you need to see the child to determine the right dosage?

How does it work?" I asked him.

"No, there's no need for a visit to us or the doctor. We calculate it based on the child's weight."

"So, approximately, how much will it cost me? Gabrillian weighs 16 kilos."

"For a child weighing 16 kilos, it would cost around 218 dollars plus shipping fees and would give you enough of the 5 supplements recommended for muscular dystrophy, for about 2 and a half months."

***

"How is your son these days?" Todd asks me.

"He's sick at the moment. The naturopath who is following Gabrillian has decided to provide supplements to boost his immune system because he constantly gets lung congestion and asthma-like bronchitis."

"Excessive mucus is a common issue in children with a Selenium deficiency and chronic cough or asthma is due to a lack of Omega 3 and 6 fatty acids. Has he had a sweat test?"

"What's that?" I ask.

"It's a test performed on children with chronic lung congestion. It measures the concentration of chloride in sweat. Pulmonary congestion can sometimes be due to an undiagnosed case of cystic fibrosis."

I looked up the symptoms described for cystic fibrosis and was surprised to see that many of these symptoms were similar to those that Gabrillian experienced.

Todd reassured me and said that even if the result turned out to be positive, they'd had cases like this before and after only 3 months on Youngevity supplements, the test showed a negative result, thanks to the Selenium intake. The conversation then took a different direction as I explained Gabrillian's various progress, such as him starting to climb stairs by himself and becoming calmer.
Todd showed me a photo of his son, who was about to turn 4.

Knowing that Todd had a child who was healthy was very encouraging.
I explained that I had recently changed Gabrillian's diet.

"It's a gluten-free diet with a low glycaemic index. Our naturopath recommends avoiding bread and no brown rice because it irritates the stomach lining. it's a high-protein diet with animal proteins at almost every meal. He also explained the importance of chicken bone broth for his joints and bones."
"Being on a gluten-free diet is one of the first requirements of the 'Dr Wallach Youngevity Program,' along with avoiding carbonated drinks, fried foods and cooking oils."

"Is Youngevity Selenium easily absorbable and does it also contain iodine?" I asked Todd. Gabrillian's physician noted that he had a thyroid problem.

"The protocol includes all essential minerals. Youngevity Selenium is the most absorbable form; it's in the form of chelated amino acid," Todd told me.

***

I learned a lot from my internet conversation with Todd. The mentality of "Defying Muscular Dystrophy" is about defying obstacles and problems, knowing that as soon as we decide to overcome these obstacles, there are always solutions available to us.

Todd's example is striking.

***

List of supplements recommended by Todd Harrison for Muscular Dystrophy:

- Beyond Tangy Tangerine 2.0
- Osteo Fx Liquid
- EFA Plus
- Ultimate Selenium
- Liquid Gluco Gel

***

July 2017. Skype call with Dr Raj.

"Since I started giving him this remedy for the pineal gland, Gabrillian hasn't been sleeping well. He has nightmares every night. Should I reduce the dose?" I ask.

"That's strange, normally it should have the opposite effect. It's a mixture that stimulates the pineal gland and the production of serotonin and melatonin, so it should also help him sleep. Continue giving him the same dose and see if it changes. How is everything else going?"

"He's still making progress physically. School is not easy, though, with his special diet and the teachers keep complaining about him. They say he's difficult and steals other children's snacks."

"You'll find ways to help Gabrillian at school too." Dr Raj reassures me. "Keep being firm at home. If he wants to eat cookies at school, it's his choice. At home, it's different, you have control. You're too soft on Gabrillian. It's not a criticism; I'm very soft with my daughter too, but her mother is strict. There are certain candies she can't eat and she just doesn't eat them."

"But I do punish him. I take away a toy." I say defensively.

"How long do you wait before giving it back to him?"

"A week, sometimes." I say.

"Try a month. Take something he really loves and you'll soon see if he listens to you."

I would later learn that in not setting clear boundaries for your child, especially from 0 to 3 years old, you are not properly educating them and also damaging their brain. Children need guidance and this is something we can see very clearly in animals, as well as in the learning of walking, of hunting, grooming and danger.

Finding a balance between an overly structured education that deprives the child of creativity and overly lax guidance that harms the functional development of the child's brain has been a long journey for me. It has meant dealing with my own emotional blocks, as a mother. Most of the time, when I didn't respect this balance, it was either because I felt guilty for Gabrillian's condition, for not being present enough for him, or because I felt overwhelmed, tired, obliged and pulled in one direction or another.

The solution was to work on and control these emotions and behaviours and to be 'selfish' sometimes.

I started setting aside time for myself. Twice a week, I go for yoga and Pilates.

I listen to motivational audiobooks every day, for at least an hour. I change my diet; no bread, reduced gluten in my diet; and no dairy products. I start feeling lighter and I have more energy. I ask Vassilis to take care of Gabrillian one evening a week and go dancing with Krasimir. I am expecting our child and later, when my pregnancy is too advanced, we go to the cinema. Every day, I look at myself in the bathroom mirror and said to myself, "Clementine, I love you. What will make you happy today?"
It's so rejuvenating to do something for yourself, something that makes you happy! Sometimes it is going for a swim in the sea, going for a coffee alone or reading a book.

Gradually, I can channel my emotions, be more centred, balanced and create enough distance to choose my attitude and the way I talked to Gabrillian, finding the right words to explain to him.
"Mom, Dimitri hit me! And he said he's not my friend anymore!" Gabrillian tells me, pointing at one of his schoolmates.

"Did you hit him too?"

"Yes."

"Then go and apologise to him."

Gabrillian comes back and tells me that Dimitri wouldn't forgive him.

“OK, Gaby” I say, “You did your duty. You admitted your mistakes and apologised. You can't control how others react because it's their choice, but you can control how you feel by correcting your actions, as you just did. Don't you feel better now?"

"Yes," he says, smiling.

CHAPTER 9
Shane Wolf's Testimony

***

Shane Wolf sent me the following testimony about his son Matthias, who has muscular dystrophy genes that have not manifested themselves, thanks to the use of dietary supplements.

"Matthias Wolf, my second son, was diagnosed with Duchenne muscular dystrophy on February 23, 2017, at the age of seven months. He was born on July 23, 2016. Our early diagnosis was a blessing for my wife and me because it gave us time to plan for our son's future. Two approaches presented themselves: following the well-established centralised approach of the standard of care or considering decentralised alternative approaches outside the traditional standard of care. We did our research (which is ongoing) and chose the latter approach. It's an approach of true hope and optimism." He writes. "My older sister Amy was diagnosed with DMD, so she was tested to see if she was a carrier of the DMD mutation. In the 1990s it was determined that she was a carrier. That's why we had our two boys tested at an early age. Interestingly, she was told not to worry about passing this on to any potential children because by then, a cure would have been found. Well, here we are in 2021 with no cure, although the Muscular Dystrophy Association (MDA) has been promising a cure for 70 years!

The MDA was founded in the 1950s and the doctors we've worked with follow the "standard of care" recommended by this organisation and its associated doctors. It's a bleak outlook. We were told that our son would lose his ability to walk and that his internal organs would eventually fail. We could hope for the opening of a clinical trial that accepts his genetic mutation and maybe a miracle would occur before his death. In the meantime, we can put him on steroids to help improve his ability to walk, for maybe six months. Well, that's simply unacceptable to us, with a child showing no signs of DMD at the time." He continued. "We were not comfortable giving our little boy powerful drugs with many side effects and very few benefits, especially when we discovered many natural remedies with visible and almost immediate results, without the side effects. Our research opened up these five possibilities:

www.doctoryourself.com/dystrophy.html. The concept of Genetrophics.

1. The supplement regimen used by Harrison and Dr Joel Wallach
2. Reflex therapy - Clémentine Ynna.
3. Stem cell therapy and Ryan Benton.
4. Ayurvedic medicine shows promise.

The website Doctoryourself.com created by Andrew Saul introduced me to Genetotrophics (Dinner Table Heredity) by Roger J. Williams PhD. This work explains that muscular dystrophy can be a geneticotrophic disease and therefore treatable, even curable or preventable, if detected early enough. This is our hope and the path we have chosen for treatment."

After reading this article, I continued to research and set up my own protocol based on the suggestions made during this research and I discovered Todd Harrison and Joel Wallach. They have already integrated this protocol into some of the supplements sold by the Youngevity company.

Todd Harrison is a man with Becker muscular dystrophy and a man who did not accept the traditional treatment model for this disease. Todd found Dr Joel Wallach and the company he founded that is based on the Genetrophics approach. These people have developed a protocol to treat this disease and Todd is getting some very positive and measurable results. Every child who uses this protocol sees almost immediate results with no side effects. Matthias has been on this protocol since we discovered Todd and started buying these products. Matthias takes a daily liquid multivitamin called Beyond Tangy Tangerine and Ultimate Selenium. The supplement ingredients are provided below. Matthias is getting stronger and shows no signs that DMD is weakening his body. We would like to add more fats like cod liver oil, high-quality protein shake and coenzyme Q10, for example. It's a long journey, which leads us to discover what produces positive results and what a five-year-old child would be willing to eat. We focus on Beyond Tangy Tangerine and Ultimate Selenium and we try to add from this foundation.

The other three treatment protocols are on our radar and we continue to learn and discern what the best options are for us on this journey.

We benefited from early detection, which gave us time to decide which approach was best for our son. Too often, parents are devastated by this diagnosis and forced to make a decision very quickly and recklessly about the path to take. I encourage parents to step back and treat all available options as Clémentine and I did with our children. The traditional model may not be in your best interest, but only you, the parent, can make that decision. We chose the alternative path and follow the doctors and patients who are getting real measurable results that have benefits with almost no side effects and we could always go back to the traditional treatment model. But, conversely, we couldn't start with the traditional treatment and then go to the alternative treatment.

Our attitude through this life experience is one of hope and optimism, not death and destruction. We will continue to learn more and adjust our treatment plan as new information becomes available. We won't give up. We will keep fighting in faith, not in fear."

"In rereading the testimony above, I noticed that it seems so easy and logical to pursue this alternative approach. So why do so many parents not choose this option? I think it's fear and the intense emotion of having your baby 'condemned to death'— or at least that's how it seems, by the muscular dystrophy association and the medical community. This intense emotional state devastates parents and we just want help and clear answers. The answers provided by the medical community and many doctors, therapists and support groups and the path they present, are very easy to follow and most of the medical expenses are covered by state insurance.

All doctors and people in the MD community are doing their best and truly care about their patients, but I believe they are using the wrong tools, i.e., steroids and getting terrible results. For example, most of the kids I see on steroids are overweight and are not an example of a good quality of life.

Finally, this path requires constant adjustment and learning about what is best for your child as they grow. It will also require undertaking some expense, on your part. Nutritional supplements can be expensive, for sure. Large support groups and doctors have no idea what we're doing and don't understand anything beyond drugs and clinical trials. They put their hope in gene therapy while we put our hope in genetotrophic therapy."

In Summary: Key Takeaways from This Chapter:

- **Keep an open mind, focus on solutions, think outside the box and look beyond scientific labels that hide the true nature of the problem.**
- **Seek the root cause of the disease.**
- **Research if others have already found the solution, perhaps written books about their journey.**
- **Believe, even if you feel naive and until proven otherwise, look for clues that point in the same direction and support this new idea.**
- **Selenium needs to come in a stable form with necessary cofactors like Vitamin E, Zinc, Copper, Chromium.**
- **Omega oils need to be encapsulated to avoid contact with air, rancidity and oil inefficiency.**
- **To be effective, the person following Dr Wallach's protocol must avoid sodas, gluten in all forms, fried foods and cooking oils.**
- **Avoid Prednisone, which increases Selenium deficiency, which can lead to DNA damage such as chromosome breakage.**
- **Excess mucus is a common issue in children with Selenium deficiency and chronic cough or asthma is due to a lack of Omega 3 and 6 fatty acids.**

CHAPTER 10
Neuro Reflex Therapy

***

May 2017

It has been four months now since I started stimulating Gabrillian's face and scalp using the Neuro Reflex Therapy technique and I have already noticed changes. He is calmer. He sleeps better. Lone Sorensen's online courses have taught me how to stimulate the frontal lobe for the activation of motor nerves used for moving our arms, leg and fingers as well as activities like bringing a cup up to the mouth and writing. It's also good for calming hyperactivity. At school, they have stopped complaining constantly about Gabrillian's behaviour and they no longer mention appointments with the psychoanalyst. Previously, every day his teacher would complain. "He can't sit still, he can't stay seated, he doesn't listen, he disrupts the class with his attitude. We don't know what to do; you need to talk to him! "

I heard the same thing every day. I even tried to punish Gabrillian, but nothing worked, actually it made it worse because he entered a vicious circle of anger with himself.

I felt exhausted and I didn't know what to do anymore. They are talking about bringing a psychologist to school to evaluate my son. Maybe they'll want to move him to a different class. Even the after-school day-care didn't want him anymore. They told me there was no more space, but I didn't believe them. We had already argued several times about Gabrillian's behaviour and the food they served in the cafeteria.

Then one day, Gabrillian's teacher said to me, "I want to talk to you!"
What had he done now? I braced myself.

To my surprise, she explained that Gabrillian's behaviour had changed - for the better!

"Gabrillian is making a lot of effort. He can sit still now; I have to remind him and ask him to look me in the eyes, but now he listens."

I listened, tears in my eyes. I was so happy. I told her that Gabrillian was taking homeopathy and I had started stimulating his neurological system.

"I don't know what you're doing, but it's definitely working!" she said, smiling.

Gabrillian has also chosen a hand to write with now. Previously, due to his muscle weakness, he would switch hands as soon as one got tired. It was something that occupational therapist Georgia had pointed out to me and had tried to correct with different exercises, like writing on a chalkboard to create an extension of the arms. That's how I realised that his nervous motor functions in the upper body, were also affected. I also remember doubting the motor capabilities of his arms after the assessment by a very prominent Israeli doctor who had come to the 'Kivotos' rehabilitation centre in Cyprus to offer his expertise. I had called him after his evaluation and he had explained to me that Gabrillian also had muscle weakness in his arms.

"My son has been examined by neurologists, physiotherapists, occupational therapists and none of them mentioned muscle weakness in the upper limbs," I said on the phone.

"I understand your surprise, but I can assure you that if you ask your son to lift his arms while creating an external rotation, you will see that he is not capable of doing it. This is a clear sign of muscle weakness in the triceps."

I hadn't paid much attention to that until the occupational therapist mentioned it again and the neurologist geneticist Dr Violetta at Makarios Hospital in Nicosia suggested the same. I remember her supporting the idea that Gabrillian also had an issue with his arms. She had also recommended that we test his heart condition. At that point in our consultation, Vassilis had reached the end of his patience and stormed out of Dr Violetta's office, claiming that she didn't know what she was talking about. On the drive home, there was a deafening silence in the car. But I had also noticed an issue during Gabrillian's swimming class. At the time, I was working at the Columbia Hotel in Pissouri Bay and with the approval of the manager Vilmante, I had arranged a service exchange with Vlada, the swimming teacher. A back massage when he had pain, in exchange for a swimming lesson for my son on Saturday mornings before the spa opened.

***

"Gabrillian, listen to what Vlada is saying! Put your hands together, extend them and then turn them."

I observed my son. He seemed incapable of extending his arms and simultaneously turning his hands outward. I remembered that we had been constantly arguing about this for months.

"Come on, Gabrillian, you're going to colour this drawing and I'll help you. Mrs. Valentina told me that you're not doing your homework at school and that you're not listening to anything!" "But mom, the teachers always ask me to colour, I don't want to, I don't like it!" Gabrillian had replied obstinately.

Now, however, I had to hide all my papers or he would colour on everything!
"Mom, look at what I drew for you!" Gabrillian said, handing me a drawing.

"Who is it?" I asked, surprised to find something recognisable in Gabrillian's drawing.

Usually, I hesitated to give my opinion on how good his drawing was because I was afraid of hurting his feelings. It usually looked like scribbles that a three-year-old would do.

But now I found I could decipher his drawings.

"It's us, look, there you are, next to Krasimir and me!"

I could discern three people, a man and a woman and a smaller child. I could clearly make out hands, arms, legs and feet.

Previously, I had noticed that although he drew legs for all the figures, he omitted to draw his own legs and feet. I also know that drawing is the language of the subconscious. Did he unconsciously or consciously omit this detail due to his disability? I wondered.

In this picture, however, I was glad to see that all his limbs, his arms and his legs were there in the drawing.

Perhaps it was a revealing sign of a change in perspective. Lone described, in her classes, how patients even experience a change in dynamics during their dreams, so deep was this work. In any case, when I was a student, I was taught that drawing a tree without its roots, was indicative of a person's unstable and fragile state. Psychologists often use drawing to understand children and sometimes adults too.

I look at Gabrillian's drawing once again. All the characters are holding hands, smiling, a sun is illuminating a sky veiled with thin clouds and in the distance, is a rainbow.

CHAPTER 11
Our Mind Can Heal Our Body

***

July 2017

Krasimir was in Bulgaria for the entire month of July. I am seven months pregnant and today, Gabrillian is with his father because it's the weekend.

I am sitting at a table on a lawn facing the sea. I love this place; it's simple, wild and full of children running around barefoot. For me, this landscape is a true source of inspiration.

I'm deeply engrossed in reading a book by David R. Hamilton titled "How Your Mind Can Heal Your Body." Dr Hamilton is an expert on the biochemical effects of visualisation on the human body. He previously worked in the pharmaceutical industry for four years after obtaining a medical degree. Now, he travels the world, conducting seminars and workshops to help people heal themselves through the power of their minds.

In his book, David Hamilton explains how to harness this power for healing. His patients also describe the visualisations they have imagined daily, to facilitate their healing.

It's fascinating. One person with a goitre—an enlarged thyroid gland—describes how, after just one meditation, Visualisation led by Dr Hamilton for a group, the size of the thyroid returned to normal proportions. He recounts his surprise and how astonished his family was at his sudden healing.

Dr Hamilton also provides advice on what type of Visualisations are most effective.

For instance, one of his most important pieces of advice is to avoid creating a war or opposition within the cells of our own body, even if they are cancerous. He recommends a more tolerant approach, such as asking cancer cells to "leave now as they are no longer needed" or to "erase inflammation with an eraser."

One of my favourite Visualisations, which I've used for Gabrillian, involves picturing the defective gene on the ground as if it were injured and picking it up, cradling it, nurturing it, giving it attention and showing compassion.

Little by little, the gene becomes stronger and before long, it joins the group of DNA.

The light of DNA then sparkles and the disease fades away.

***

Visualisation for Muscular Dystrophy

Ah, there's a little boy and a little girl on the lawn! They're probably at about the same age gap as Gabrillian and my future baby, Julia. I'm observing the little girl's first steps. She's very excited and prefers to run to maintain her balance. Her brother is as cheerful as a lark, running around her, jumping on the bench and the chairs.

At that moment, I visualise the healing of my son.

I nurture, protect and feed his DNA and his muscles strengthen. I imagine the muscle fibres starting to push, the motor nerves beginning to function.

I then imagine Gabrillian's thin, fragile legs and his slender quadriceps. Now I see a weak muscle with no energy, poorly irrigated due to his posture and the condition of his joints. His nerves are not functioning well.

I enter his nerves and move up to the spinal cord, into the spinal cord and then up to the brain.

The frontal and temporal lobes of the brain are overloaded with information, perhaps because Gabrillian has an above-average IQ, he is also hyperactive and speaks three languages. I also notice a blockage in the part that separates the two hemispheres of the brain, the part responsible for coordination and balance.

I also see dysfunction in the master glands like the hypothalamus and the thyroid gland due to the constant contraction and tension of the neck muscles, which also impede proper brain irrigation. Just mentally moving through these different areas causes new nerve and blood flow in these different parts of the body.
I also see an accumulation of toxins causing blockages in the brain, coordination problems and issues in the intestines that are not receiving enough stimulus.

The pelvic muscles and diaphragm also seem quite weak, preventing proper inflation and expulsion of air in the lungs.

The liver seems overloaded due to Gabrillian's poor digestion and elimination, leading to an accumulation of toxins and mucus, sources of inflammation in the body. The liver is not functioning well and not producing the necessary chemicals for good muscle tone.

I then go deeper into my son's liver cells until I see the proteins, enzymes and finally the DNA of the cells. I see the defective gene, all curled up by itself. I have compassion for this fragile little being. I take it in my arms, cradle it and at that moment, the gene gradually fades and I am drawn inside, as if by a vacuum.

Inside the DNA is like a starry sky where the stars represent the protons, neutrons and electrons.

I then head towards the source of these atoms. I imagine entering an immense space of complete tranquillity and I see a large, very peaceful lake.

I then ask Gabrillian's body to show me the waves related to his illness and suddenly large waves appear, gusts of wind sweep through my hair and over my face, drops of rain trickle down my face and in the distance, lightning spikes out of large grey clouds.

This landscape is both fascinating and terrifying.

With a firm yet gentle voice, I shout "Stop!" and suddenly the waves disappear, the sky is calm and starry again and the lake seems to have fallen asleep.

I realise that I have just cancelled Gabrillian's disease. Now we will emit new waves by throwing a stone into the lake. Each stone generates a certain colour representing our intention, as well as a certain vibration.

I choose green for vitality, health, youthfulness, nature and its therapeutic effects.

I add blue and a new wave appears on the water's surface. This blue is penetrating, calming and represents tranquillity and balance.
A pinkish-red wave appears that I associate with vital energy, the warmth of good blood circulation and the proper functioning of the body.

The orange colour that appears next, is a sign of light and vitality. Each colour adds new attributes to Gabrillian's body.

A violet wave sweeps over the others, signifying transformation and acceptance of the present moment as well as forgiveness.

I gradually move away from this scenery and find myself outside this unique space, contemplating an aurora borealis in a sky tinted with beautiful colours.

I am once again projected outside, tumbling over and over, until finally I find myself outside Gabrillian's body.

I ask Gabrillian's body, "Show me that it's done!" All the colours appear around my son's body and undulate with perfect grace and fluidity.

I know it, I feel it within me! The change has occurred!

I thank the Universe: "Thank you! The work is done! The work is done!"
My eyes well up and I now see not a little boy but Gabrillian jumping and running.

It's such an intense experience and I am so happy because I know deep down that Gabrillian is healed.

***

I remember that at that time, we were awaiting the results of Gabrillian's EMG, which, according to Dr Manel, a neurologist at the Mother and Child Hospital in Lyon, was supposed to confirm juvenile spinal atrophy type 1 or 3. She was so sure it was the correct diagnosis that she had not even requested any additional tests.
The results arrived sometime later and to our surprise, Dr Manel announced that they needed to conduct further examinations because the results were negative.

I was intrigued and so relieved that Gabrillian wasn't going to have that label. I then remembered all the Visualisation exercises I had done and wondered, could it be that this has blurred the lines and changed Gabrillian's reality?

Mira's voice came to mind: "You know, Clémentine, in metaphysics, the past, present and future are one. There is a reality where Gabrillian has a deformity and a higher reality where Gabrillian is perfect, running. If you can bend these realities and make them converge, you can change your destiny - and his."

We wanted to travel to Bali. I remember thinking, "What's the point of being here if you can't be present with your children? What's the point if you can't enjoy the present moment?" The mere revelation of this thought was a shock to me! I made an effort to be fully present, to enjoy the little moments and to appreciate them.

Every morning, I would list all the things I was happy and grateful for in my life, starting with the beauty, good health, my children's creativity, all the way to the different flavours and colours of my breakfast, not forgetting my cosy duvet and pillow that allow me to dive deeply into restorative and revitalising sleep, for all the cells in my body.

Every time we went for a walk, I practiced being present. I sat on the beach and tried to feel all the sensations of fresh sand under my feet, the pressure points of my feet on the ground, the tickling of the grains between my fingers, the refreshing smell of the sea breeze, the touch of Julia's cold hands on my neck. And every time I felt my mind drifting elsewhere, I reminded myself: Clémentine, come back to the present!

One day, we were walking by the sea and I thought to myself, "I'm already in Bali!" A week later, we booked our tickets to Bali! The best part was that once in Bali, I realised the importance and simplicity of being present because Bali is so enchanting, like a walking meditation.

I realised that all the self-work had trained and prepared me to be a match for the experience I truly sought in Bali.

Finally being present for myself and my children was so nourishing!

***

Later, I met Joyce, a holistic shamanic therapist, at a women's circle in Cyprus. "You are a very strong woman, you know, because the universe never gives anyone something they are not capable of overcoming," she told me.

This sentence resonates in my mind and I remember the photo hanging on my success board on my wall (a success board is a poster where you stick photos of things you want to manifest in reality).

I had a photo of the Maasai tribe who are known as the warriors of light. The Maasai have such faith in the universe that when they encounter an obstacle, they celebrate their victory because they know the universe is just and it only gives them challenges they are capable of overcoming. They are confident and grateful for this gift and they know this new adventure promises new spiritual growth.

***

The Meaning of Life

According to the words of a spiritual woman, Nicola, whom Mark had introduced me to in England, it would seem that in one of his past lives, Gabrillian had been my mother and had rejected me because I was a handicapped boy.

"Interesting," I thought to myself. Perhaps we have swapped roles today to understand our mutual attitudes better? Maybe this experience allowed us to put ourselves in each other's shoes to find the deeper meaning, understand each other's actions and words and draw a great lesson from it. It was, in fact, the perfect place to truly forgive each other.

This is something I also experienced in this life when I got together with Krasimir, after my separation from Gabrillian's father. Sometimes I let Krasimir argue with Gabrillian about something he was still too young to understand. I didn't say anything, I didn't intervene. Maybe I was afraid of asserting myself and jeopardising another relationship! And then I thought, "This is not good for Gabrillian to see us arguing and disagreeing."

I recalled my stepmother arguing with me and sometimes it felt unfair, but my father said nothing.

Now I was in my father's place and I understood his point of view and I forgave him for not always intervening. Because what I had taken as abandonment was, in fact, his way of maintaining our family's balance.

I would certainly never have understood that if I hadn't had this experience.

I understood that Gabrillian's disproportionate and clumsy body had taught him to have more empathy and compassion for others.
I also understood why I tended to get upset when Gabrillian was clumsy because I saw myself in him, I felt my own frustration, having been clumsy and rejected myself. So now I was much more aware and every time I was about to get angry, I remembered why and was able to calm myself.

It was also a way for me to gain perspective on what was happening with Gabrillian's father. Many times, he didn't pay proper attention to Gabrillian's diet and eventually, our son would get sick. Initially, it drove me crazy to feel so powerless about the situation and our son's well-being. And then, gradually, I realised that everything is a process and Gabrillian's healing is a journey that only Gabrillian can choose to undertake. So my response was to let go of all that control that would only make the situation worse and to continue to inform and educate Vassilis and his family—let go of control and accept what it was. This idea calmed me down a lot and eventually, things started to change.

Vassilis began to be more involved and he now gave Gabrillian fresh chicken or rabbit every week, eggs from mountain-raised hens and freshly caught fish.

Vassilis's mother even occasionally did Dr Raj's massage for Gabrillian.

In the end, acceptance and forgiveness were a significant transition for me towards Gabrillian's healing because you cannot give what you do not have.

I spent most of my childhood navigating between shame, constant humiliation and anger towards my family and circumstances like my mother's death and wanting to make them pay, to finally standing up to all those who looked down on me. Finally, I understood that I needed to forgive if I wanted to be free to evolve and reach acceptance and finally, the peace that could heal me from all my emotional traumas. That in turn would allow me to heal Gabrillian. Forgiving implies taking responsibility for what I allowed myself to accept and what I let pass through me.

Would the humiliations at the table have had the same impact on me if I hadn't internalised at some point that I was not 'as I should be,' that I was stupid and that I didn't deserve to be there?

The universe was just reflecting my own thoughts back to me and all these experiences only emphasised and justified my initial doubts about my worth.

The path to healing begins with self-work because I cannot be a guide towards acceptance for my son if I have not worked on myself.

"When we are no longer able to change a situation, we are challenged to change ourselves."

Viktor Frankl, Man's Search for Meaning

***

Creating a Vision

"Mom, why can't I run like the other little boys?"

I knew that this question would eventually come my way, but I didn't expect it, not right now.

"My dear, you are unique and after all, you can jump and you can also run now. You have everything you need!"

I decided to create a Vision Board with Gabrillian.

A Vision Board is a board where you place images, photos and affirmations related to what you want to create in your life—your goals, ambitions, dreams.

What you'll need:

- **A board or an A3 sheet**
- **Coloured markers**
- **Magazines with topics that interest you**
- **A pair of scissors**
- **Glue**

"Gabrillian, what would you like to do? What would you like to do more often?"

"I want to do Kung Fu, swim with my dad and go on a cruise!" So we cut out pictures from magazines of a child doing karate and wrote underneath: "Every day, I become stronger and stronger."

I asked Vassilis to take pictures of them both at the sea and after printing them, we glued them onto his A3 sheet.

I then asked Gabrillian, "How do you feel when you swim with your dad?"

"I'm happy; I love my papaki (the nickname he had given his father); I feel free."

So we wrote that, underneath the photo. In another magazine, there was an offer for a cruise to the Greek islands. Gabrillian said, "I love boats, Mom and papaki does too!"

"Visualisation is one of the most powerful mind exercises you can do. According to the popular book 'The Secret,' 'The law of attraction is forming your entire life experience and it does so through your thoughts. When you are visualising, you are emitting a powerful frequency into the Universe.'

Whether you believe it or not, we know that Visualisation works. Olympic athletes have been using it for decades to improve performance. Psychology Today reported that the brain patterns activated when a weightlifter lifts heavy weights are also activated in the same way when the athlete just imagined (visualised) lifting weights."

Excerpt from Huffpost: https://www.huffpost.com/entry/the-scientific-reason- why_b_6392274

CHAPTER 12
We Are On The Right Track

***

Skype Call with Dr Raj, August 7, 2017

"Hello Clémentine, how are you?"

"Hello Dr Raj, I am fine, thank you. We just returned from our trip to France for Gabrillian's muscle biopsy."

"Please keep me updated on the results when you have them." Dr Raj said.

"Yes, of course. Gabrillian also had staphylococcus infection on his leg, three times! The doctors and dermatologist recommended giving him antibiotics, which I did, reluctantly. I am now giving him Mangosteen juice."

"That won't work. These types of parasites are primarily located in the nose and ears and will come back. I'm going to tell you what to do. The Bac-Tox remedy is the one for these kinds of bacteria, you will give it to him in a litre of water with Solidago and Carduus (these are remedies for the liver and kidneys), to help elimination. You are also going to give him a massage twice a day and give him the chicken broth I recommended, twice a day. Once a week, you will rub him with Hibiscrub which you can find in pharmacies."

I jot down his advice in my notebook.

"Gabrillian's father always gives him sweet things, I don't know what to do, I have told him so many times, but he just won't listen to me. Also, he refuses to do the massage for Gabrillian although sometimes his grandmother will do it."

"Please give me his number again, I will arrange a Skype call and explain the importance of the diet and massage." Dr Raj says sternly,
"I've noticed that Gabrillian gets tired very quickly when he eats and he has vomited twice." I said, "It was more bile than anything else. He will say that he is tired and can't eat anymore." I notice Dr Raj's worried expression, but he quickly recovers and says:
"You will now avoid giving him nuts and seeds although nut butters are still good. No grains such as rice and quinoa, no dark-skinned vegetables such as tomatoes, eggplants, peppers or potatoes. Also avoid fruits and not too many vegetables either. Focus on green vegetables such as spinach, Swiss chard, etc., which are easier to digest. Also, blend the vegetables and put only a few small pieces of meat in the soups for him to chew. Give him eggs for breakfast and occasionally gluten-free porridge. Twice a day give him chicken broth with meat or fish and a few green vegetables. If you want to cook a dish with flour, I recommend using buckwheat flour."

"Can I use odourless coconut oil, the one that does not have a very strong taste and is not always enjoyable with every dish?" I ask.
"Yes, that's fine, you can use that."

"And instead of sugar, what do you recommend? Stevia?"
"You can give him cinnamon, that's very good, or a little Stevia but not too much."

"What do you think of agropyrum powder, wheatgrass, or maca?"

"You can give them to him occasionally as green juices, but not in smoothies with fruits as they contain too much sugar. I don't really recommend these kinds of powders because they are dry and dehydrated and can prevent absorption and block the digestive system, so please don't overuse them."

Dr Raj continues: "Give him quality meat to nourish the muscles with good proteins, this will be especially helpful for Gabrillian."

I nod and say, "A few days ago I noticed that Gabrillian had blood in his stool, is this something I should be concerned about?"

"Gabrillian must have been constipated before and it's possible that the stool dislodged a piece of inflamed mucous membrane in the anus."

"Should I use salts or montmorillonite bentonite powder in Gabrillian's bath?" I ask.

"No, don't use anything else."

"I also noticed that Gabrillian very quickly switches from hyperactive behaviour to a very phlegmatic, tired type behaviour."
"Every time Gabrillian eats something that doesn't suit him, like gluten or sugar, it's like he takes a hit to brain becoming uncontrollable and then very tired." Dr Raj explains.
"OK, I need to be even more careful about what Gabrillian eats. When do you think we can start the heavy metal detoxification?"

"His digestive system must be perfect and after that it's very easy with cilantro and chlorella."

Dr Raj nods. "The whole world is wondering how to get rid of heavy metals and most go too fast. We are on the right track, keep it up."

CHAPTER 13
Birth of a Little Sister

***

Gabrillian's little sister arrives on
September the eighth, 2017

In my hospital bed, I am well settled, a pillow behind my back, earphones in my ears listening to various interviews about brain rehabilitation.
"Hello!" says the duty nurse. "How are you? Do you need any medication, anything?"

"Hello!" says another nurse and I remove my earphones automatically. It must be the tenth time someone has come to check my blood pressure.

It's starting to get dark. Tomorrow morning, very early, I am scheduled for a caesarean section and I must admit that it worries me a bit.

However, it's not the same as the first time with Gabrillian. Now I have tools, I have done all my breathing exercises, my stretches and now it's time to listen to a meditation by author Louise Hay ('Love Yourself') to help me relax.

I've written all my fears in my journal, everything that's going on in my head, for fifteen minutes. It's healing and soothing to name all these fears and now I feel empty and light.

I also reformulated in my journal my greatest fears and added affirmations such as "Success is mine, all the time," and "I am safe in the universe".

In studying the very foundations of ancient Chinese medicine, one learns that man is a microcosm of the universe (the macrocosm) and by definition, every man or woman contains all the energy of the universe. That's a powerful affirmation, isn't it? We also learn that energy never disappears but can sometimes be blocked in certain energy channels called 'meridians'.

I think back to those autistic children, whom Lone Sorensen, a specialist in rehabilitating disabled or autistic children, explains have energy blocked inside the internal meridians that regulate the excesses of other meridians. According to Lone at some point, these children reject their external environment and turn inward and by doing so, they lack nerve impulses to vital organs— such as the digestive organs—creating all sorts of problems.

I start having contractions and they become more and more frequent.

I hesitate. On one hand, I want to have my baby naturally but on the other, if I start giving birth, they may take me directly to the operating room and an unscheduled caesarean section is not the best thing, from what I've been told. I would be put under general anaesthesia and I understand waking up is very painful.

"Come on, I'll wait a bit longer." I say to myself.

In my wait, I start receiving different information. I see these autistic children and their energy blocked in the meridian vessels and suddenly the image overlaps with one of Gabrillian. I get the idea that it might be the same for my son, all these learning difficulties, his poor eye contact, his hypo and hyper-sensitivity. Is it just a matter of blockages?

I also remember the words of William Doré, the creator of a "Brain Gym" technique, who explains how stimulating certain parts of the brain can improve balance and coordination. He is convinced that it is a matter of the effect on the Cerebellum. To have consistent results, it is necessary to stimulate the Cerebellum repeatedly and he also talks about specific exercises to stimulate different parts of the brain.

My contractions are now very close together. I decide to call the nurse.
I do my breathing exercises. In my mind, I review the yoga exercises and start by focusing all my attention on certain parts of my body to soothe them. It gives me a sense of control and I doze off a bit.

Then everything happens very quickly. They came to get me for the caesarean section. This time it goes well. I explained my previous traumatic experience to the nurse and she took good care of me and then finally, Julia is here.

"When are you going to bring Gabrillian?" I insist.

"Aren't you tired? Don't you want to wait a few days and rest a bit?" Vassilis asks on the phone, a bit surprised.

"No, I want to see him now, he might be a bit disoriented, he hasn't seen me for a week."

"OK, I'll ask my mother to bring him.”

Gabrillian is very excited; he has brought a little pink unicorn for his sister.

"Yaya, look, she's moving!" Gabrillian says to his grandmother.

I also receive a congratulatory card from Yaya and we talk while Gabrillian plays with the controls of my hospital bed.

"Gabrillian, calm down!" I look at my son, he's holding the support bar and swinging on it as if he were Tarzan.

After some time, Gabrillian leaves with his grandmother. I watch him from the balcony of my room. I am sad. I feel like I haven't really spent any time with him. Also, I notice that his behaviour has worsened. He is more hyperactive than usual and he loses focus. "Gabrillian, bye-bye!" I shout from the balcony.

He hears me and turns around. He is delighted.

"Mom! Yaya, look! It's mom, over there!" he shouts. His grandmother waves to me and I hear her tell Gabrillian that it's time to let me rest and that they will come to see me soon. Gabrillian keeps turning back to wave goodbye; it's as if he's afraid I'll disappear. I feel his fear and it breaks my heart. He has always been afraid that something will happen to me or his father. I remember the time I was sick on vacation. He stayed with my parents and when he saw me, on the phone screen, lying on my bed, he was so worried. It was the same every time we went on vacation in France and his father stayed in Cyprus; he cried constantly. He also repeatedly told Vassilis, "You want to see me for a long time, right? Then stop smoking, dad!" The fear of death is ever present for Gabrillian. He asks a lot of questions about it.

Then I hear in my head the words of Suzanna, Gabrillian's physiotherapist. "It's going to be a big emotional shock for Gabrillian, the birth of his sister. You are one of the loves of his life and you've spent all summer with him," she told me. Gabrillian is a very emotional child and every strong emotion creates many physical symptoms for him. For example, if I scold him and he feels guilty or scared, he starts to cross his legs in a chaotic way. It's as if he loses all sense of coordination and of course, then he loses his balance and falls. He also loses all sense of time and ability to make eye contact, or he reacts in a totally disproportionate way by starting to cry, shake, or even say that his heart hurts. It can be quite an impressive display, but I think there is some degree of manipulation as well.

Julia, my new-born, begins to wake up and I return to my room to take care of her.

I remember that the universe only gives the opportunity for us to accomplish and take responsibility for what we are capable of and because of that, I will find my way and my balance.

Being armed with patience and self-love and not allowing myself to fall into guilt or paranoia, that's what I need. I know the way now because I've already taken it.

With a smile on my lips and a new light in my eyes, I approach Julia, kiss her on the hand and whisper to her: "You, I am sure you came to earth to help Gabrillian and me and with your brother, you will be the best friends!”

CHAPTER 14
Third Visit to London

***

Visit to Dr Raj in London, November 2017

"Look at me, mom! Look what I can do!" says Gabrillian, who is as excited as anything.

We have stopped at Pinner Park. In an hour we have an appointment with Dr Raj.

Gabrillian shows me how he can now run and walk well. It is true that his gait has improved a lot. I was a bit afraid that after the arrival of Julia, because it was such a big emotional shock for him, he had started to stutter and often cross and uncross his legs.

I was so worried about his sudden lack of coordination that I talked to Suzanna about it.

"Yes, I've noticed too but I don’t think we should worry too much about it at the moment because Gabrillian is a very sensitive little boy and there's a good chance it will pass on its own."

It's true that little by little he started to improve, especially since I also treated him with Neuro Reflex Therapy sessions to his face using a technique created by Lone Sorensen.

Gabrillian has found a small lake with lots of ducks. I give him his rice cakes to crumble and throw to the ducks. Gabrillian is in heaven. He has always loved contact with animals. "Well done, my chick. Come on, now we have to go," I coax him away.

"Hello, Dr Raj!"

"Hello, Clémentine, hello Gabrillian! Oh my, I can see immediately that he has made huge progress! Look at the way he walks!"
"Yes, Gabrillian's physiotherapist is very happy with his progress." I am delighted at Dr Raj's reaction.

"And you, Clémentine, are you happy with his progress?"

"Oh yes, of course!"

"Now it would be good to work a little more on his hip movement," says Dr Raj, carefully observing my son's gait. Gabrillian starts to undress, ready for Dr Raj's massage.

Dr Raj invites him to sit on a stool in front of him.

This is the only time when Gabrillian is more or less calm because he loves Dr Raj testing him with the bio resonance machine.

"Gabrillian is doing much better," Dr Raj tells me.

"What is that red line?" I ask.

"That represents his thyroid gland. I'm going to prescribe something for that!"

Dr Raj prescribes the remedy 'Thy- Tox' for Gabrillian. On Google, I read that it is a homeopathic remedy specifically designed for detoxification and repair of the thyroid, parathyroid and pineal glands. Autoimmune thyroiditis (Hashimoto's) is the most common cause of an underactive thyroid. Wheat gluten has been shown to be a trigger for Hashimoto's. Selenium deficiency, a serious problem due to low soil levels of this mineral. Selenium deficiency leads to suppression of the conversion of T4 to T3.").

"Gabrillian is doing much better overall, however, he still tends to have congestion in the sinuses, bronchi and lungs."

I see from Dr Raj's expression that he is a bit concerned. He tells me that he will also give me something for that.

He will prescribe liposomal vitamin C, based on Camu Camu. It's a very strong complex that will nourish and repair the immune system and adrenal insufficiency. It is thought that absorption is multiplied 5 times as it bypasses the liver and intestines, which seems wise, knowing that Gabrillian has leaky gut syndrome! He constantly has digestive problems—constipation or diarrhoea—he gets tired very quickly, he has skin problems. Are we working on Gabrillian's leaky gut problem?" I ask.

"Yes, that's right!" Dr Raj confirms.

I remember when I described all of Gabrillian's symptoms to Dr Raj and he told me he saw a lot of potential in Gabrillian, I had known that he specialised in leaky gut or candidiasis problems. The results of the electro-acupuncture only confirmed his suspicions by seeing the state of the spleen, thymus, intestines, thyroid and adrenal glands.

This Camu Camu-based compound also stimulates the brain and the production of neurotransmitters.

"Just give him the tip of a teaspoon every day," Dr Raj advises me.

"Does he need to take probiotics again?"

"Yes, he needs them."

Dr Raj prescribes 'Energetix Flora Chewable' which is composed of vitamin C, Chicory root and Lactobacillus sporogenes probiotics. "What do you recommend for his behavioural problems, his hyperactivity? I also notice that he had difficulty learning. I tried to teach him the numbers up to 20 in French and even with a strong promise like permission to play on the iPad for half an hour, it took him two days and interactive stimulation with songs to remember." I tell the doctor.

"I prescribed this for you. Be careful with the dosages, they are very high. It stimulates the brain, the pineal gland, the pituitary, hypothalamus and the limbic system."

I would later learn from Lone Sorensen that the limbic system is the reservoir for all our negative emotions and experiences. It acts as a protective system, very useful in prehistoric times to avoid being devoured by predators although obsolete today.

However, with the media continuously directing our attention to wars, viruses, thefts and murders and with the hypersensitivity of children like Gabrillian—the limbic system gets overloaded. These children are constantly flooded with disturbing information, often unconsciously, by parents who have become completely desensitised to this kind of data and do not see the danger.

"Also do this massage, but be careful, only in the evening to calm him down."

Dr Raj shows me a new manipulation. He presses the inside of Gabrillian's thigh while checking his pulse.

I film what I do to make sure I don't miss anything.

"I took a course in Neuro Reflex Therapy, do you know it?" I ask him.
"Yes, I know it and it works!"

"I'm going to Oman at the end of February, as a volunteer to educate families on how to treat their children using this technique, under the supervision of my mentor. Do you know Lone Sorensen, she's the specialist who created the 'Sorensensistem' method?"

I had started studying Neuro Reflex Therapy Sorensensistem when I was pregnant with Julia, I had come across it by chance in a YouTube video. Lone, the specialist explained how this therapy had cured her son who was born with a rare syndrome. She had also lost all hope in traditional medicine after spending months in the hospital with her son, Christian. Her son suffered from multiple seizures. The doctors kept giving him new medications but the seizures just got worse.

Lone said that it suddenly came to her. She thought, why not try reflexology? After a few months of working on her son with reflexology and homeopathy, Christian was doing much better. It took him a few years to be cured completely but today Christian is a completely fulfilled family man.

"You can see testimonials and videos online about this method," I added.

"I don't know Lone, but I take care of the Sultan of Oman. I go there often. When you go, take this with you, it will do Gabrillian good!"

Dr Raj hands me a box. “It's Frankincense from Oman.”

"I love the fact that you want to help other people, Clémentine, that's great!" Dr Raj encourages me.

"Why don't you patent your massage method and offer training?" I ask.

"I already do," Dr Raj says, I have students who come to study here."
"I would really like to learn your method. How long does it take?" I ask.

"It depends on the person, but generally it's quite a long process. The massage and homeopathic protocol are different for each individual. I start by educating parents about the diet to follow. The most important thing is to be very good at using the bio resonance machine and evaluating imbalances with it. Wait until your baby grows a bit and then you can come here for training and you too, little Gabrillian, you will come to study and help others." Gabrillian is now super excited.

"Would you be willing to come to Cyprus to help other children like Gabrillian if I organised a 'detox retreat' for children and adults with muscular dystrophy?"

"Yes, of course, with pleasure!" he says.

"Could we organise an interview in the near future to explain your method to other families who would benefit?" I ask.

"We'll wait until we have more results, Clémentine. Not now but later, yes. If you gather a group of parents, I will talk to them and explain. We could even arrange this online because I also have parents in the United States who are part of our group."

"That's a great idea!" I am genuinely excited.

Gabrillian is messing around in Dr Raj's office because he hasn't been getting attention for a few minutes.

"Gabrillian, come here! Stop touching everything!" I shout. "Do you have other cases with behaviour like my son?"

"Yes, of course and some much worse, by the way! I have worked with many children with neuro motor diseases. Let me show you a little boy I treated in India. He couldn't walk but after just a few weeks of massage, now look at him."

I watch the video.

I can't believe my eyes when I see the difference. This only confirms my choices! I'm on the right track!

"Of course it's cerebral palsy, it's much simpler and faster than working with a child who has muscular dystrophy, like Gabrillian." "Your therapy actually works on another microsystem than Lone Sorensen's Neuro Reflex Therapy on the hands, feet and head, doesn't it?" I ask. "I noticed that you treat the left side more than the right, is it because it's the lunar or Yin side, that will work on the parasympathetic system and have a sedative effect on the corresponding organ? To balance the spleen for example, which seems to be Gabrillian's biggest problem? I understand that with Neuro Reflex Therapy it's different, there's a regulating effect that works on both the right and left sides, you can't just work on one side because it unbalances the organ and because the brain reflects both sides."

Dr Raj nods. "Yes, my technique is different and there isn't just one Yin and Yang, right and left of the body, there are actually many on the human body. When we have time, my colleagues and I look for new ones," Dr Raj said, enthusiastically.

"In Gabrillian's case, you're working on the leaky gut problem first, aren't you? How long do you think it will take?" "It depends on the person and their level of involvement.

Gabrillian is already doing much better, maybe it will take about a year in total."

The receptionist hands me a paper with a list of newly prescribed remedies and explains how to use them. Dr Raj walks us back to the front door. Gabrillian is very happy because I have promised him lunch in a restaurant.

Gabrillian's eyes are shining, he knows that the wheel is turning for him.

***

December 2017, in France

"Gabrillian, come here!"

The people in the waiting room look at me as I start to get impatient. Gabrillian, of course has found the loudest toy, rolling it from one waiting room to another. 'Crrrrrrr' goes the little car. A mother asks him if he can make a little less noise.

The doctor arrives.

"Gabrillian and Clementine?" the doctor asks, surprised and annoyed not to find Gabrillian in his examination room. It's 4 pm and we've been at the Grenoble University Hospital Centre (CHU) with my father since early morning.

The secretariat informs us they will contact us as soon as the results are in.

After several hours of waiting, Dr Testard, a paediatric neurologist, enters the hospital room.

"Hello, how are you? How is Gabrillian? Did everything go well?" he asks my father and me.

I say that Gabrillian is fine now.

"Gabrillian, come here, little one!"

Dr Testard observes his walk and confirms that Gabrillian has made progress since the last time, although he seems to have distal amyotrophy in his calves as well.

I explain that although Gabrillian is making great physical progress, he seems still to be affected at school, his teachers constantly complain about his attitude.

"It might be advisable to have him tested for ADHD, he seems to show the signs. It's usually hereditary. Have either you or his father been diagnosed? It's not very serious but these are children who generally have difficulty integrating into a group and making friends."

Memories rush through my head.

"Clémentine, pay attention! You've got your head in the clouds."

"Hey, Clem, where are you going?!"

Difficult times from my childhood resurface and the common thread of all these events is my total absence, as if I had disappeared into my world, markedly isolated from other children. Sometimes I felt so different that I would do anything to get noticed and be loved and tried to make that happen with my good grades.

And it's a tendency that I find in my son, he always tries to be liked by other children.

Dr Testard leaves and informs us that the hospital's occupational therapist will also visit Gabrillian, in an hour. Gabrillian watches cartoons from his hospital bed and I take the opportunity to dive back into my book bought a week earlier at Fnac in Lyon: "Journal of a Food Intolerant".

Captivating and so true, it also contains lots of little tips. I want to give a little talk about food, food intolerances.

The truth is, it's not easy to follow and even less so to limit one's child.

We don't realise it, but eating is really an act of belonging and integration into society.

And when you don't share the same tolerances as most others, the simplest family outings, snacks at school, meals in the cafeteria and afternoons at the beach can become really chaotic. How many times have I found Gabrillian sitting waiting for me, watching other children eat cheese pasta that he is not allowed to eat but loves so much?

I had found a way to organise myself and come to pick up Gabrillian to eat at home bringing him back to spare him the sight, but sometimes I was a little late.

As a parent, it breaks your heart every time there's a birthday at school and the teacher calls you and asks if Gabrillian can eat a chocolate cake.

And there I am at work, I can't bring him a gluten-free or sugar-free cereal bar to have as a treat along with the other children. Also, it's not the same because Gabrillian does not share what other children eat or do and again it sets him apart.

Gabrillian wants so much to be integrated and play with other children that he has even started to be influenced by some belligerent children to win their sympathy. And then, the teacher calls me and tells me that Gabrillian hit another little child, he pulled down a little girl's skirt. When I ask Gabrillian why he did that, he explains to me that

"It's Dimitris, it's Stelios who told me to do it."

I was so tired. On one hand, Gabrillian was getting better, he was making progress and on the other, it was getting worse. In France, I had found the book "Journal of a Food Intolerant" by Margot Montpezat, in which she describes her story, how frustrating it can be sometimes, to be gluten intolerant, how cruel people can be and how she finally found her way.

She also underwent psychological therapy and shares interviews with experts on the subject in her book.

The food psychologist interviewed explains that, more than the deprivation and its physical side effects, a diet is not trivial at the psychological level. He explains that eating is a social act and can also be a taboo subject.

Reading this book did me a lot of good, to hear the perspective of someone intolerant, to put myself in Gabrillian's shoes and ultimately to discover that there are solutions.

Margot describes the best way to apologise for what we cannot eat, without offending our hosts, is to ask at a restaurant for a 'gluten-free', sugar-free and dairy-free menu.

You empathise with her when she is teased by her family, her friends and when her loved ones accuse her of exaggerating, saying that it's all in her head.

You feel her frustration when she is offered cheese tagliatelle, knowing she cannot eat it.

You feel close to her when she spends an hour in organic stores deciphering all the labels of different products and ultimately having to put most of them back because products are labelled "gluten-free" when they contain cheese or butter, or "sugar-free" but contains aspartame, which is carcinogenic.

Margot also explains the culinary differences of different countries and their dietary advances. In the United States and the United Kingdom, for example, they are very advanced.

In London, you will find “Gluten-free” options in most decent restaurants and some also encourage the consumer to let them know their allergies or food intolerances for a tailor-made meal. This is not really the case for France, even in Paris where restaurant owners will give you a dirty look if you dare ask for an alternative to traditional bread or cheese.

The French are so proud of their traditional ways.

The island of Tahiti, the birthplace of the author, is a paradise for lovers and consumers of coconut milk and gluten-free products. This is not always the case for these exotic countries. When we went to Bali, you would think that with all their coconut trees they would cook only with coconut milk, but no, they cook everything with butter!

Margot also gives alternatives for milk, butter, cream and gluten with examples of her own recipes.

What also pleased me was to hear from someone else's mouth that blood tests do not show all allergies and food intolerances because I probably had to repeat that at least fifty times to Vassilis!

***

Krasimir and I got married on December 27, 2017, at Paphos Town Hall.

A new chapter in my life opens up for me, with a man who loves me. I am happy.

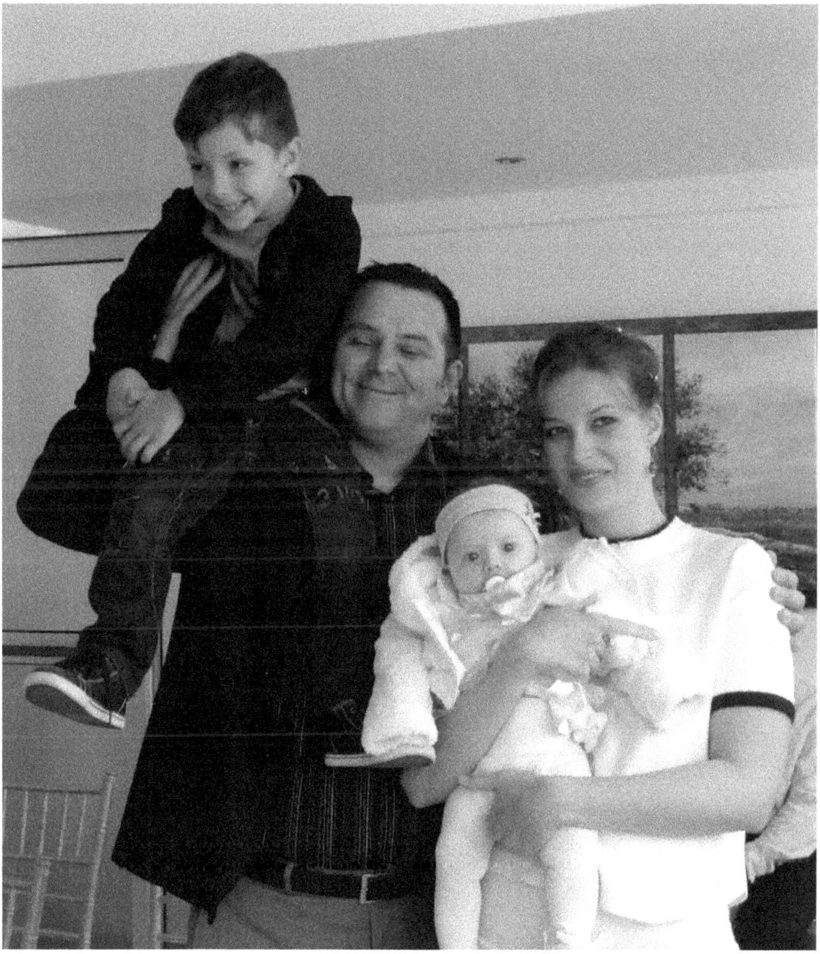

CHAPTER 15
Trip to Oman

***

February 2018

Here I am embarking on a new adventure, going to the desert in Oman to help families, parents and their children.

I had completed my training in Neuro Reflex Therapy, received my diploma and had already started working with very interesting cases such as people suffering from multiple sclerosis and high blood pressure, with some very good results.

Neuro Reflex Therapy is a technique that includes both Aboriginal and Oriental practices, as well as cutting-edge neuro-anatomical research.
It is based on the latest research in neuroplasticity—the ability of nerves and brain cells to regenerate.

We work on the face, on 'reflex zones', neurological points that activate the production of nerve messengers and stimulate certain parts of the body, an organ or the brain. This technique is also known as 'cyber therapy'. It's a bit like our brain is a computer and the neurological points are a keyboard. It is thus possible to open certain "software" and to correct their content. This correction is only possible by treating the primary cause of the dysfunction—in 90% of cases, it's an emotion that created an avalanche effect and led to the body's imbalance. We also activate with the sharp side of the thumbs on certain scalp—lines that correspond to certain structures of the cranial box—to stimulate blood circulation and spinal fluids in different parts of the brain. This stimulation allows for the regulation of certain fluids called humours, such as blood, lymph and cerebrospinal fluid.

On the feet, we press certain reflex zones defined by traditional Chinese reflexology and a neurological zone corresponding to the spinal column. Thanks to this technique, it is possible to regulate posture by releasing all nerves under pressure and by adjusting the column a bit like a chiropractor but working with the reflex zone instead of the spinal column itself.

This method also allows activation of what are called dermatomes, meaning that different parts of the skin but also different organs, glands, structures and muscles are connected to different spinal nerves. That means it's possible to treat different organs by pressing on the reflex point of the corresponding spinal nerve.

On the hands, we also have a large number of nerve endings corresponding to certain organs and to the hips, shoulders, etc. We also use Korean neuro reflexology based on the discovery of more than 100 meridians.

Hands are also very effective for regulating hormonal problems. More than the effect on physical symptoms such as fatigue or hot flashes, hormones are responsible for our mental state like anxiety or behavioural problems. Indeed, if our brain is not nourished with the substances it needs, different behaviours will be generated. This is the case with children who have muscular dystrophies because this is an important component of the brain and often leads to behavioural problems such as ADHD, ADD or chronic anxiety.

However, neuroplasticity is only possible through repetition, as this creates new neural pathways and new behaviours and abilities.

One day I came across a video of a Bedouin family in Oman with three disabled children, all unable to walk. Lone Sorensen and her team had gone to the desert to train the family in a method called Temprana. It's a method based on the latest research in neuroplasticity. The family had to manually stimulate three areas of the body, the face and skull, the hands and the feet.

I watch the video and can't believe my eyes. After 6 months, the two children aged 6 and 10 start to walk and the 21-year-old starts to crawl!

I think to myself, "I have to go there and discover this rehabilitation system! I want to meet Lone and see what she is capable of, I want to immerse myself in her mindset!" Shortly afterwards, I receive an email from Lone about an upcoming expedition to Oman. She needs volunteers to train families with children who have brain problems. Only therapists who have already obtained their diploma in Facial Neuro Reflex or Temprana can apply. I see an opportunity and apply!

***

I say goodbye to Gabrillian and he asks me if I'm going to the land of camels!

I kiss Julia, my 5-and-a-half-month-old baby. This is the first time we will be separated. My heart is heavy. I whisper in her ear, "Mommy will be back soon, you'll see! And if leaving you for ten days at such a young age teaches you later to pursue your dreams to the end, then I will have succeeded in my role as a mother! I will miss you a lot!"

Gabrillian has escaped to his room. He doesn't want to talk to me, he's waiting for his Yaya.

I explain to him what I'm going to do, that I am going to help little children like him, learn a lot of things, follow my dream, but I can see that he's not very receptive to my words. I then promise him a surprise from Oman and his eyes immediately light up.

***

"Hello, Clémentine!" Lone says to me with a smile.

"How was your flight? You are the last one for tonight. Let's go into the room."

I look at Lone. It's very strange, I feel like I know her. Maybe after all those hours studying facial neuro reflexology on my computer screen, I know her voice and her expressions so well. Lone Sorensen is the director and founder of the International Institute of Reflexology based in Barcelona, Spain. Lone was born and studied in Denmark and she also has Argentine origins and offers her courses in Spanish as well. She is a pioneer of Neuro Reflex Therapy and Lone has also focused on helping disabled children or those with special needs. She will develop a technique called Temprana Reflex Therapy specifically for this purpose. Temprana means 'early rehabilitation' and aims to intensively and specifically stimulate a child or adult.

This method consists of stimulating neurological points and creating new accelerated neurological pathways, maintained with the contribution of another technique called Brain Gym.

"Brain Gym" activates the Pons part, located between the two hemispheres of the brain and promotes the creation of new neurological pathways. Co-ordination is favoured by stimulating the right and left hemispheres of the brain.

I had decided nine months earlier to pursue this training in Facial Neuro-Reflexology because of the benefits of this technique on concentration, improvement of learning and reduction of hyperactivity.

I was immediately passionate about it. I knew reflexology was an effective method, especially for things like pain, sinusitis, etc. And then one day, while I was massaging Gabrillian's feet in front of one of his cartoons, it came to me like a flash. What if I could help him, with reflexology?! After all, he really enjoyed the foot massage.

I had forgotten this idea and hadn't thought about it much. But the more I learned about this technique, the more I was impressed by the depth of Lone's research.

Lone explains the case of her son who was born with a rare disease. He has no hair and has many epileptic seizures. After days spent in the hospital with doctors who keep giving her son new drugs that only worsen his condition, she quickly becomes disillusioned with the medical approach. She comes up with the idea of treating her son herself with foot reflexology. After a year of reflexology treatment combined with homeopathy, her son recovers 100% of his faculties and no longer has any seizures.

After a few years, Lone decides to move to Argentina and open a clinic there.

She tells the story of a young girl with a very unsteady gait and muscle spasms. "I want you to treat me yourself, please," the young girl says to her.

Initially Lone is bewildered. She has never treated such a dramatic case before. She asks for help from colleagues and begins to work with new techniques applied to the face. The first time she works on the young girl, all involuntary muscle spasms disappear. When I hear this story, it catches my attention. This technique must be very powerful.

Lone also recounts how she learned this technique by watching for hours as Andean aborigines massaged each other. “This technique was mainly taught to the women of the tribe. Often the older ones would massage the younger ones at a specific time each month. If they were injured, men sometimes resorted to this therapy as well,” Lone narrated. Lone drew numerous sketches and maps mimicking the aboriginal processes and back at her institute, with the help of other therapists and doctors from her team she researched to find correspondences with other known systems and microsystems.

The research proved extremely interesting and they discovered a new very powerful system corresponding to the central nervous system.

"You will meet some members of your team tomorrow because for our friends from Australia the journey was very long and they have gone to sleep." Lone told me in the taxi.

We arrive at a sort of farm and I am shown to a very large dormitory. The living room is adorned with long benches in the style of ‘One Thousand and One Nights’, with a huge chandelier in the middle.

I share the room with Shermine who is of Lebanese origin and lives in London and an Australian, Bobbie, who has Polish origins. I meet the other volunteer neuro-reflexologists the next morning at breakfast.

Cathy is from Melbourne, Brigitta is German and Lissy and Anne Marie are from Denmark, like Lone.

Late in the morning, we start our lessons on theory. We sit under a patio. It's hot and the little breeze and iced hibiscus tea cool us down a bit.

Lone tells us many patient stories to give us context and also teaches us her techniques in a less conventional way. I immediately appreciate the fact that Lone's courses teach by illustrating very telling examples, taking us into her world.

Always having been passionate about ancestral medicine, I find myself in a group of very well-educated people, sharing the same admirations and aspirations.

Lone begins to tell the story of the three children from the Oman desert with muscular atrophies. I hang on her every word.

"The children were from a very poor family that was sponsored by the Sorensen Institute. They are a family of eleven children, three of whom suffer from a syndrome that causes muscular atrophies. Of course, under these conditions, there was no certain diagnosis due to the cost of analysis and the distance from the city. However, with our examination technique, we don't need a diagnosis because it is possible to feel, manually if there are blockages in the nervous system of certain organs, glands, or systems."

"The three children were born that way and none of them could walk when we started therapy. They could move their upper bodies because only the lower body had been affected. The eldest also didn't speak and was a bit autistic. We trained the family, the three older sisters, to work on them every day. After four months, when I returned I couldn't believe what I was seeing! The youngest was now able to walk! Subsequently she was also able to run and it was a great joy for me to see all the new possibilities that were now open to her. The second, who could not walk before, was now able to stand for a short period.

He was also able to take a few steps. Of course, when we started he was already 14 years old and this was progress over only four months." Lone explained.

"It's important to know that the earlier the therapy starts, the better the results." Lone tells us, "The eldest was now much, much, much less autistic. I noticed it immediately because I could make eye contact with him. He was also now able to walk on all fours. And this made a huge difference to the family because you can imagine this 21-year-old, sitting in his corner, whose only pleasure is to eat and who is grossly overweight as a result with his father, a very thin man, having to carry him to the bathroom. That's very hard. Many people don't know what it means to have a disabled child. And there in the desert, as a toilet, they just have a hole in the ground outside, away from the house, with some boards around for privacy. It was to this makeshift toilet that his father had to carry him! It's a very difficult situation! Now the young man could walk on all fours to the toilet, to his bed and come and eat with the rest of the family and he had also lost weight. If I remember correctly he lost about 18 kilos."

"I also taught them a supplement to the therapy called the 'cross crawl' that we sometimes use for the disabled who don't have access to physiotherapy and also for social autism or ADHD problems. I use two types of brain gym, the traditional American model and another less traditional one that is very different, so I have a total of 54 movements that I can use. This technique was very good for the 21-year-old Omani man to stimulate his brain and help him lose weight."

"I stayed in contact with this family for quite a long time, although I was not able to return and they informed me that their children continued to develop well. They became more autonomous. The 14-year-old started to walk for longer. Lately, I haven't had contact, however, I'm pretty sure they continue to develop well and do the therapy. The little one is certainly doing well now.

They were very good sisters, motivated and committed to helping their siblings and that made a lot of difference because it's very important that parents don't give up and that they continue therapy."

I interrupt Lone with a question.

"Lone, do you remember if these children also followed a special diet and heavy metal detoxification?"

Lone nods, "This was a very poor family and they unfortunately had no idea about heavy metals or specialised diets. These are the results of only four months of Temprana Therapy and Brain Gym." she replied.

In the months that follow, Lone and I had the opportunity to talk online, many times. Lone explained her point of view on muscular dystrophy during our discussions.

"It's a problem of chemical reaction. The liver is responsible for more than 300 different chemical reactions and the production of enzymes or proteins for the proper metabolism of the body. It is also closely linked to the proper functioning of the hormonal system. The liver is therefore responsible for proteins responsible for muscle tone."

Excerpt from PubMed

"Skeletal muscle mass loss is a major component of malnutrition and occurs in the majority of patients with liver disease. Lower muscle contractile function also contributes to the adverse consequences of sarcopenia. There are no effective therapies to prevent or reverse sarcopenia in liver diseases. This review will discuss advances in diagnosis, pathogenesis and treatment options for sarcopenia in liver diseases."

Source: https://www.ncbi.nlm.nih.gov/pubmed/26974417

Lone's second subject was motor neurons and how they function in the brain. I learned that it is the frontal part of the cortex that is in charge of all body movements and more particularly the prefrontal cortex which would give the signal.

The decision to stand up, for example, starts from the prefrontal area and then the impulse goes from the central nervous system protected by the spinal column to the muscles. A second part called the 'motor sensory cortex' located at the back of the frontal part of the cortex, also comes into play. This part of the brain coordinates motor and sensory nerves and that's how I learned that the function of walking is also a sensory experience.

Lone explains that just like swallowing saliva or going to the toilet, walking is only possible with the functioning of these two parts of the brain, being a motor and sensory function. For example, children with Asperger's syndrome walk on tiptoe because unconsciously they don't like the sensation of putting their foot completely on the ground.

I also learned that significant neurotransmitters are located in the large intestine, hence the importance of a perfectly functioning digestive system for treating brain dysfunction or mental problems. Knowing that Gabrillian has leaky gut syndrome, it seemed quite logical to me that he would also have motor nerve dysfunction issues. The proper functioning of the hormonal system is also closely linked to the colon, knowing that if one gland is in disharmony, it inevitably leads to a disorder of the other glands as all need to work together. However, major glands such as the pituitary, pineal and hypothalamus located in the brain, are responsible for the production and command of all other glands, much like the conductor of a musical concert.

And guess which materials are most sensitive to heavy metals? Yes, the brain and the glands!

Gabrillian was also diagnosed with a thyroid gland issue. The thyroid works closely with the adrenal and sexual glands. Lone also teaches us that children with brain dysfunction or damage often have respiratory and digestive problems because they do not receive nerve impulses to the organs, muscles of the diaphragm or digestive tract.

Gabrillian often has asthmatic bronchitis and has also been diagnosed with nasal polyps, which were resolved after a year of Neuro Reflex Therapy and daily intake of Frankincense extract, from Oman.

***

Temprana Reflex Therapy

We arrive at an institute specialised in treating autistic children in Muscat, Oman.

After visiting the institute, Lone gives a speech to explain what Temprana Reflex Rehabilitation Therapy is.

"We are here to explain what Reflex Therapy is. I work with children with different problems, not only autistic but also ADHD and with various other syndromes.

With this therapy, it is possible to create a specific protocol for each brain problem or for an organ or a system. I have been working in Oman with disabled children for 8 years and I came today with a team of professionals who work in different countries. I am also the founder and director of a school, 'The International Institute of Reflex Therapy' where I have been teaching Reflex Therapy for 40 years. I have various international educators around the world, like Mohammed in Jordan, who train professionals interested in my technique in their respective countries. The only place where I work myself is in Oman. We are also in the process of opening a school here." Lone says.

"My method is based on the principle of intensive stimulation at home. We train parents to treat their children at home. I think you know the importance of intensively stimulating such children otherwise there are no results. It's a method by which it is possible to change the behaviour of the brain, thanks to its neuroplasticity."
Lone points to different parts of the face, reminding us that certain parts of the face are linked to certain parts of the brain called 'reflex zones'. It is therefore possible to change the behaviour of the brain by stimulating certain zones or reflex points on the skull, hands and feet.

"I could also work on the whole body, but I have devoted my research to these 3 areas: head, hands and feet. The evaluation takes place in different stages and the first stage is observation. I observe the child, I can detect attitudes and I will also listen to the family's story, how the birth went, the pregnancy and what happened with the child."

"What kind of questions? What do you ask, for example?" one of the educators asks.

"Questions about the pregnancy," Lone says, "whether the mother took strong antibiotics during pregnancy or at the time of delivery. Many women have an infection in the uterus and if the child swallows this fluid it can generate encephalitis, for example. In a long and difficult delivery, the child can be affected emotionally as well as suffering the effects of lack of oxygen. Children become autistic because they are always on the iPad or other tech. Humans develop with movement and if a child does not move, they do not develop well.

There are also children who become autistic after vaccinations. Some, completely brain damaged. And it's not a question of what I think, it's what I've seen with my own eyes." She says.

"Here, in Oman, there's a phenomenon that my team and I call 'Omani TV Syndrome' where children are in front of the TV all day! From eight months, all day in front of the TV! From the earliest age, which are so important and on top of that, they are fed formula milk! Any child would become stupid with this regime. I have already had 23 cases like this. The children have no language, they have no eye contact and are totally hyperactive!"

After the lunch break, Lone continues.

"So, how does Rehabilitation with Neuro Reflex Therapy work? First of all, I analyse the different neurological points, the reflex zones on the face, on the feet and I can feel the blockages. There's a different feeling, what we call different deposits, different degrees of tissue rigidity, which give me information about the nature of the problem, the severity of the problem and where I need to focus my work. And that's how, without needing a previous diagnosis, only with what I see with my eyes and what I feel with my hands, I am capable of creating a protocol adapted and specific to each child.

I search manually for certain zones on the face, you can see, in the documents handed out, the different colours for different zones. All brain dysfunctions are capable of being stimulated and regulated by stimulating different reflex zones. This is what is called a 'micro system'. If you can imagine a map of the brain present on the face, feet and hands.

This is only possible with the neuroplasticity of our brain and our nervous system—which gives the possibility to modify a child's brain. If this was not possible then your work as a special educator, occupational therapist or physiotherapist would make no sense. You too modify the brains of children."

"Is this neuroplasticity only possible with autistic children, or applicable to other cases?" one of the educators asks.

"Of course, we also work with children who have attention deficit, various syndromes and paralysed children. We have children who were autistic and who end up not being autistic at all. This is very different, of course and varies from child to child."

"So, what are the steps? First, I will organise a protocol and then I will train the parents. For example, for a program with an autistic child, the training takes place in a day, or two or three. Three days of training is more for children who also have brain damage. Then, the family will go home and the parents or other family members will perform the treatment three or four times or in some cases even six times a week.

And at that point, we have two different cases—one where the parents regularly and conscientiously perform the protocol and they get very good results and another case where parents (and unfortunately this is often the case) do not perform this work and therefore see no results.

For example, one 12-year-old boy, in just 3 weeks showed enormous positive changes. It depends on the families. It must be the case for you too, I'm sure. You have families who have the energy at home to support your work and others who don't. It's a very easy tool to use, we only use our hands." Lone holds up her hands. "We just need a little coconut oil for example, which is very practical especially if they are living in the desert like some families I have trained. The educators at the institute seem very interested and more than once we demonstrated the techniques used on them."

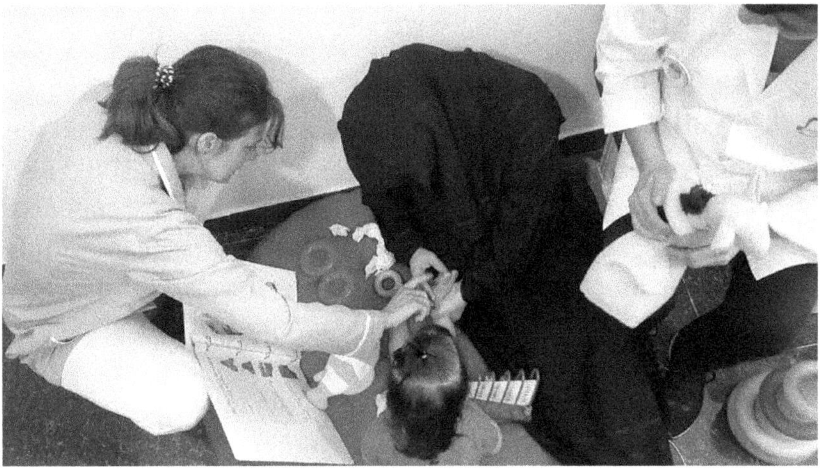

Clémentine, training a family in Oman with Lone Sorensen and a team of neuro reflexologists.

***

During my stay in Oman, I encounter a striking example of this work and the results it generates.

Omer, son of Aisha, head of rehabilitation in Oman, is a 14- year-old boy. He suffered from cerebral palsy due to encephalitis when he was little. His mother did not give up on him, as the doctors had recommended. In search of solutions, she discovered Neuro Reflex therapy and eventually she and her sister were trained in the Temprana method.

Today, Omer no longer has epileptic seizures, he walks with a slight sway, he is capable of having an interesting conversation and speaks English and Arabic fluently.

At the end of my trip to Oman, Lone hands me a green folder. "Here, Clémentine. This is the Temprana protocol I prepared for your son."

A few days earlier, Lone had asked me to make a list of all Gabrillian's symptoms. This list includes:

- A waddle-like gait reminiscent of a duck's.
- Muscle atrophies in both thighs and weakness in the calves and triceps (for the calves and triceps, it could also be amyotrophies, but only Gabrillian's quadriceps have been scanned using MRI—magnetic resonance imaging)
- Weak lungs, chronic congestion, recurrent sinusitis, very dry nose, coughs a lot, takes Ventolin (doctors explained that this was due to his weak pelvic muscles which couldn't expel all the mucus from the lungs)
- Weak trunk, very loose abdominal belt (since his esophagitis as a baby and his constant crying, his belly remained swollen and loose)
- Hyperlordosis still flexible and a non-fixed scoliosis.
- Knee and elbow hyperextension (he is hyper lax, like me), with ankle problems, feet turned outward.
- Leaky gut syndrome, frequent diarrhoea. Food intolerances.
- Sugar intolerance.

I reread my list and suddenly I realise that all this seems much more manageable than the medical diagnosis of "muscular dystrophy" and "there is no cure."

Upon my return to Cyprus, I am enthusiastic and impatient to try this new protocol on Gabrillian.

After everything I saw in Oman, the functional recovery of children, all the stories told by Lone and other therapists and the striking example of Omer, I am full of hope and filled with gratitude.
I pass through customs and the agent signals me to pass, I smile knowing that in my bag is a package of Frankincense resin from Oman.

I can't wait to see the effects on Gabrillian.

I arrive at his grandmother's house, who has taken care of him during my trip.

"Mama, mama!"

Gabrillian rushes up and hugs me. I kiss him on the head.

"Oh my little one, I missed you!" I say and take a plush toy out of my bag.

It's a camel with 'Oman' written on its hump and when you press its belly it sings an Arabic song in a child's voice. Gabrillian loves it. He is very happy with his gift. Arriving home, after unpacking my suitcase and kissing my five-month-old baby a thousand times, I settle on the sofa, ready to start the massage for Gabrillian.

We start with Dr Raj's massage, then I decide that tonight we will only do the head and hands because this first massage is lengthy. Tomorrow morning, we will do the feet.

I also brought an oil back from Oman that contains Frankincense essential oil. It smells so good.

Gabrillian lies on my lap and I start the therapy.

During my stay in Oman, I had the opportunity to massage Lone Sorensen and be evaluated and guided on any errors I made. "Make longer strokes," Lone says to me then, grabbing my hands to demonstrate how I can amplify my movement to cover the entire area to be treated.

"It's the hormonal system and your son needs a good stimulation of this area," she says.

I had shown her the entire procedure without forgetting the lines and points on the skull, representing the frontal lobe of the brain, for good body movement.

"Perfect, I'm impressed, you're on the right track," Lone says to me with a smile.

Her words echo in my head as I perform the therapy on Gabrillian and I feel a new confidence in myself.

I start doing the reflex zones and pressure points on Gabrillian's feet.
I am surprised to discover how many inflammations and infections I can feel in his body with my thumb, especially with the new technique that Lone had shown us in Oman. I had asked Lone why the pressures were performed upwards, as it was the first time I had seen that, even though I already had 13 years of experience in plantar reflexology.

"It's a matter of brushing against the grain, so you feel the nerve endings more and therefore feel the imbalances in the body more,"

I look at Gabrillian. Even though it seems quite sensitive, given the number of imbalances and the crystals felt under the soles of the feet, he had fallen asleep and even seemed to have enjoyed this massage.

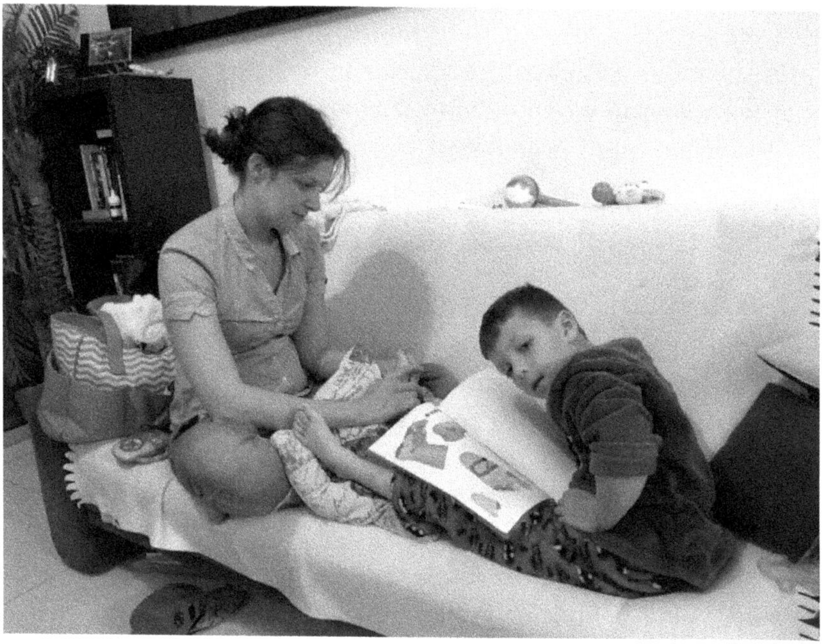

***

April 2018

A few weeks later, we decide to go for a walk. There is a walk along the sea that runs alongside a row of hotels in Paphos. We like to go there with my husband because it feels like a holiday with all the tourists lying on their sunbeds, covered in tanning oil and the breath-taking view of the waves crashing against the rocks. Gabrillian is excited, he is delighted to discover little iguanas on the walls, which he calls dinosaurs. They too bask on the rocks surrounded by masses of red and pink flowers that smell of rosemary. Gabrillian brings me a small branch and rubs his hands with it.

Before leaving for the walk, I had explained to my son that it was time for him to walk without taking the stroller. He was strong enough now and soon his little sister would also be walking. Hearing this, Gabrillian is determined not to be outdone by his little sister, so we leave the stroller in the car. I explain to him that we will stop when he wants to and we can sit on a bench. It's the technique I use when I see him getting tired. Instead of asking him if he is tired or if his feet hurt, I invite him to sit next to me.

It works very well, but if I ask him if he is in pain or tired, he starts to complain and will not make an effort to push himself because he's easily persuaded by words. "Come on, my little one, let's sit on this beautiful bench! Look, we can even see your dinosaur friends." Gabrillian sits for two seconds then gets up again. I see that he has spotted the hopscotch chalked on the pavement.

He explains to me that he knows how to play, he will show me. Two days earlier, I had seen him observing two little girls playing hopscotch and he had asked me what they were playing. Finding a small stone, Gabrillian approaches the hopscotch.

He throws the little stone and to my greatest surprise, he starts jumping from one square to another. I couldn't believe it! A few weeks earlier, any attempts to jump would be in vain or resulted in very low jumps ending with loss of balance.

Now I was watching a little boy with a lot of confidence launching himself with assurance, his jumps were about 10 centimetres high, his landing was perfect, his balance and his gait now so much more balanced and assured. Tears in my eyes, I was watching a little caterpillar that had come out of its cocoon and was now unfurling magnificent wings of ease and promise.

CHAPTER 16

Fourth Visit to London – Gabrillian's Healing

***

November 23, 2018

"Gaby, come my little one! We're going to do your workbook together!" I say to Gabrillian, handing him a book I'd bought at the airport. We have already done the sticker collages and he is proud to show me how good he is at mathematics. The special educator had mentioned Gabrillian's progress in mathematics. The pilot announces the upcoming landing and the cold weather awaiting us at Stansted Airport, England.

How peaceful this trip has been. Gabrillian has been well behaved throughout the journey.

I also congratulate myself on my new habits—playing with him and giving him more attention.

We first have an appointment with a friend I met in Oman, who by coincidence, also knows Dr Raj.

***

"Hello Shermine, it's so nice to see you again! How are you?" I turn to introduce my son.

"Your mom has told us so much about you, it's nice to meet you Gabrillian," says Shermine, smiling.

We have lunch at an Indian restaurant that Dr Raj recommended. The staff is very attentive when I describe everything Gabrillian cannot eat.

Eventually, he orders "Tikka chicken" and as he is tired of always eating chicken, I tell him it's a kind of bird, which isn't really a lie. He is excited to see Dr Raj and doesn't eat much. Soon, I take leave of my friend.

After arriving half an hour early at Dr Raj's office, we decide to go for a hot chocolate. I enter a café and ask the waiter if they have coconut milk to make a hot chocolate. After confirming that is possible, I announce to Gabrillian that he will have a hot chocolate.

"Mum, look, there's a little heart in my chocolate!" Gabrillian is excited with his hot chocolate and wants to take a photo. As he attempts that his chocolate spills on the table and the floor.

At first, I'm a bit annoyed - couldn't he be more careful?' but then I calm down. After all, it was an accident. It happens to everyone. I explain to the waiter that we've had a catastrophe. Gabrillian feels uncomfortable. He tries to wipe up the mess. I realise, suddenly how much he has changed. He is so much more responsible now and tries to fix his mistakes.

The waiter asks Gabrillian if he wants another one.

"Yes!" says Gabrillian, excited to have a second chance. This time he lets me take a photo of his hot chocolate. He drinks it in small sips, savouring his drink and after a few minutes, we cross the street to Dr Raj's office.

"Dr Raj is ready to see you," the secretary tells us. In the white corridors, all the doors look the same. I recognise Dr Raj's door by the photo of a little French bulldog on the opposite door to his office.

"Hello Clémentine, hello Gabril...." he stops, mid-sentence as he watches my son walk.

"Oh my God, look at him! He has progressed so much! Clémentine, next time keep me informed of Gabrillian's progress, so I don't have a heart attack seeing the results!" says Dr Raj, clearly delighted.

"What can I offer you to drink? A tea, maybe? Gabrillian, do you want water?" asks Dr Raj.

"We just had a hot chocolate—with coconut milk—so I think yes, a little water for Gabrillian would be welcome." I say, looking at my son. I had to constantly remind him to drink water. He could easily go a day without drinking. He holds out his plastic water bottle to Dr Raj to show him he already has water.

"We're going to give you another kind of water, you'll see!" says Dr Raj.

Gabrillian is already sitting in his chair, ready to be tested with the Bio resonance machine.

"How long has it been since we last saw each other?" He asks

"It's been a year. I've had a lot of travels." I smile.

"Yes, you went to Oman. Did you like it?"

"I did and I learned a lot."

I look at Dr Raj's screen. Most of the boxes are now yellow, which shows balance. There are no longer any red boxes that represent inflammation, infection, poor circulation, etc. "Gabrillian's thyroid gland is doing much better. The spleen is still a bit unbalanced and he also has skin problems but all in all his progress is very good."

I think of Gabrillian's recent complaints at night, complaints that he itched and I noticed that he also had eczema.

"Dr Raj, I recently bought a DVD to study a diet that had similarities to the diet you recommend, the 'GAPS diet'."

Dr Raj shook his head forcefully

"Don't do that, don't do that diet for Gabrillian! I will explain to you."
"So fermentations of cabbage, fish, all that is not good?" I ask.

"No, let me explain with a diagram. You will never forget once you understand it."

Dr Raj takes a sheet of paper and gestures for me to come closer. "Look, let's take the example of a plant, a leaf. Bacteria will start to colonise living matter if you ferment it. If they are good bacteria the living matter does not disappear. On the contrary, if the bacteria are bad bacteria, parasites, the matter, this leaf for example, will disintegrate. When you ferment cabbage, for example, you will see very well that the matter begins to decrease to make more room for the juice, which means that these are parasitic bacteria.

Now look at this other diagram: this is the digestive system with the oesophagus, stomach, intestines and colon. Everything above the intestines is sterile, so why introduce parasites into the stomach? You will cause a lot of damage this way! I had a client who followed this diet and the results were catastrophic. She ended up with huge skin problems and it took me more than a year to restore the state of her digestive system. Forget all these fermentations, kimchi, kombucha, sauerkraut, all that is not good."

"What about fermented yogurts like kefir? I have to say I digest more easily eating yogurt with my food."

"It's because you eat little of it." Dr Raj replies.

I start reading him the details of all the different ingredients and processes used in the GAPS method and the only one that seems acceptable in the context of Gabrillian's diet, is the administration of ginger tea between meals.

List of Products to Avoid

- Molasse
- Sauerkraut
- Sauerkraut juice
- Beef and fish stock - prefer chicken stock Kefir - consume little
- Goose, duck fat
- Fermented fish (mackerel)
- Pickles
- Gravlax Ghee made from unpasteurized butter

CHAPTER 17
Trip to Bali

***

December 2019

Finally, we are here! I have always really wanted to go to Bali! I had read that there they have healers who transmit their knowledge from generation to generation. It was even said that in Bali, ancient manuscripts in Sanskrit, unique to the region are preserved, which would explain why they have particular and ancient knowledge. When I asked them if they taught their technique, they told me no and that only specific families in the region possess this power.

"Mum, why do these statues look like monsters? Is it to scare children?" Gabrillian asks me as he sees a roundabout with many quite frightening statues, from the taxi window.

"If you are afraid of them you should bring them offerings so they stop bothering you," the taxi driver tells him.

"In Bali, we believe in Yin and Yang and everything is made of part light and part shadow. That's why our statues also represent it." I think, this civilisation is so different from what I know in Europe. It seems based on complete acceptance, there is no duality of good and evil as in the West. Every person has qualities and faults and we tend to show only our "good" side and hide what we think is our "bad" side. In the East, they recognise the importance of both sides which allows a certain harmony. There is also an absence of judgment, a mountain has a shadowed side and a sunny side, one cannot exist without the other. Why not accept us for who we are and only after this honesty and vulnerability, allow ourselves to change to a better version of ourselves. But first accept and see in each of our behaviours—or behaviours of others that we don't like—an opportunity to surpass ourselves and restore our balance.

"Do you never get angry, while you are driving? You drive so close to each other and you hardly ever have accidents, how do you do it?" asks Krasimir, astonished.

"We respect each other, that's how," says Mike the driver.

I look down again, I can't believe it. Gabrillian just went down and up over 100 steps in the middle of the jungle. He was excited by the immense waterfall, the biggest in Bali, waiting for us at the bottom. He was so proud to be a little adventurer. He's seven and a half. It starts raining because it was the monsoon season and after climbing the slippery steps, Krasimir, with Julia in his arms and I with Gabrillian by the hand, we dry ourselves in a small hut while we wait for the rain to stop. It was so impressive, the waterfall had now turned brown and the noise it made was both frightening and fascinating.

I look at Gabrillian. Yesterday, for New Year's Eve, instead of partying and because we were in the middle of the jungle, we took a paper and a pen and wrote down our goals for the new year.

For Christmas, we went to an orphanage. In Bali, if parents cannot pay for their children's food and education, they must place them in an orphanage.

"Can you imagine choosing between your children because you can't provide for them all?" asks Baba, an Australian living in Bali. Baba is a schoolteacher in Australia and now devotes his life to serving the children of the orphanage. He works a few months in Australia and comes back with money to feed the children and volunteers to improve the sanitary and educational conditions of the children.

"What would you wish for this new year?" Krasimir asks the children to write their wishes on a piece of paper.

We collect the papers and start to read them:

"New shoes; my parents proud of me; a schoolbag."

I watch Gabrillian who had written a PlayStation 4. He tears up his piece of paper and on another one writes "I want all children to be happy!"

I look at him and think this is a lesson he would never have learned it at school!

CHAPTER 18
Bio-resonance Therapy at Home

***

May 2019

"Mom, look what I can do!" exclaims Gabrillian with his new snorkel mask.

He is so happy in the water, the waves undulate around his body, no handicap can be seen. In the distance, I see my husband talking to his friend Galia who has invited him for a meeting. She has something important to explain to him. After a good hour of swimming, I decide to join them with Gabrillian.

"I think this is more my wife's field, isn't it, my dear?" says Krasimir in the middle of his conversation with Galia.

"Sorry?" I ask. "What's it about, I didn't follow the conversation." Galia explains to me that she had used a bio resonance machine for the past six months with astonishing results. Galia explains to me that it's an MLM (Multi-Level Marketing opportunity). I have a natural resistance to MLMs but I listen anyway. I realise then that the operation is very similar to what Dr Raj does. There is also a program for anti-parasite cures, a follow-up with a Russian doctor who is coming to Cyprus who can examine Gabrillian and create a personalised protocol.

I can also test Gabrillian myself through a program called "quick test." In just a few minutes, this program can detect any body systems that are not functioning well.

These results are 95% accurate thanks to a universal electronic system that continuously compares previously recorded databases by other operators around the world. Although the company is mainly based and developed in Russian-speaking countries for the moment, due to little effort on translation, it offers great promises for expansion.

Galia continues to try to convince me and also offers me the opportunity to try it myself, not knowing that I have already decided to buy it.

We arrive at a hotel and go up to the first floor. Gabrillian is excited. He loves tests. Dr Tatiana arrives and sets up the equipment. She does not speak English but she understands my questions and Galia translates her answers for me.

I explain Gabrillian's latest DNA diagnosis to her. Doctors in France have finally found that Gabrillian might have SMALED (Spinal Muscular Atrophy of Lower Extremities).

Tatiana starts to test Gabrillian. She begins with a quick test to see the general state of his system. At first glance, she explains that this is not a genetic disease because his "vital energy" is very strong. She continues to check Gabrillian's different systems through a database of chemical constituents. For example, she compares Gabrillian's chemical reactions when in contact with "ginkgo biloba" which gives her an idea of the state of his circulatory system. Seeing the red colour of the box corresponding to the head organs, she tells me that Gabrillian does not have good brain blood circulation. She continues with Selenium which completely disturbs his hormonal system, especially the thyroid gland. She explains that she is now asking questions to the electronic system, such as: is it genetic? The answer is no. Is it due to vaccines? Tatiana explains to me that he is positive for the DT polio and diphtheria vaccine and that the system confirms that this would be the reason for his muscular dystrophy.

She will prepare a complex for him to run overnight the next day. She hands me my "Life Balance," a portable bio resonance machine, the very next day.

I study my son's complex. It will work on his liver, his cerebral circulation, his nervous system.

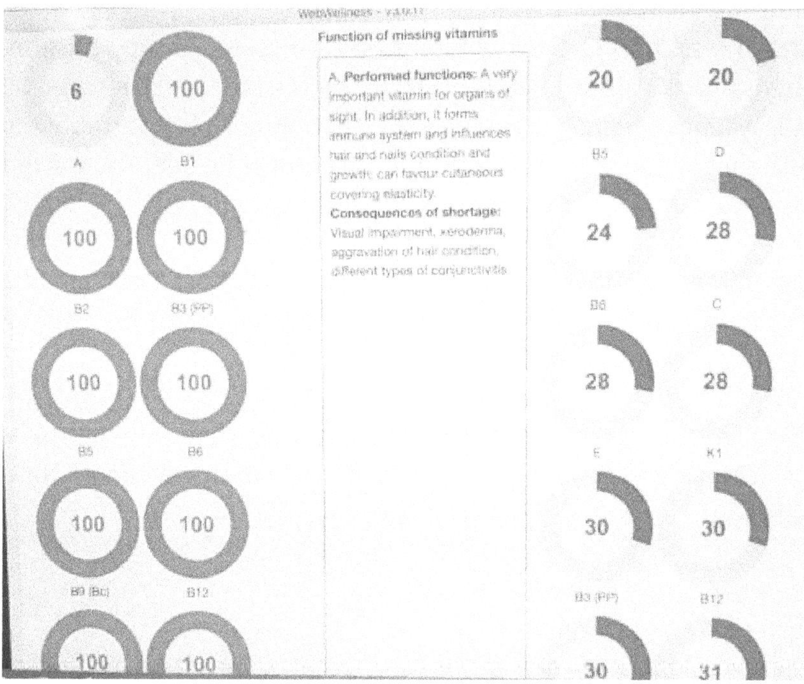

Before (right) and After (left) the therapies of vitamin absorption level and physiological state of the organs.

***

September 27, 2019

"Gabrillian is sick, Chori," Vassilis tells me on the phone.

"What's wrong?" I ask him.

"He has a sore throat, headache and he's very tired."

"OK, bring him to me, I'll do his therapy," I reply. I set Gabrillian up on the machine after giving him drops of frankincense. I place his feet on copper electrodes and give him two electrodes to hold. I attach two more around his head.

I put the TV in front of him so he's happy because after the quick test of less than two minutes, I do a 20-minute therapy for him. Then, I do his Neuro Reflex Therapy on his face and feet and he falls asleep. Finally, I download his treatment on his portable bio resonance machine and for about 45 minutes he keeps it around his neck. I do a quick test to see how his immune system is doing.

Incredible! The level of his organs, which indicated red criteria due to inflammations in his body, are now all green! His vitamin level has gone from near 0% to now 100%!

I couldn't believe it, it was so fast! I ask Gabrillian how he feels. He assures me that he is fine and asks me when we can go for a walk.

***

For a whole month, during the long COVID quarantine, Gabrillian did not go to his usual physiotherapy twice a week. We noticed that his spine began to curve more to one side, accentuating his scoliosis.

I decide to try to help him through one of the latest therapies I'd learned to correct posture. After just one session, the results were incredible, his whole spine became straighter, his posture was different, his protruding belly became much less prominent.

After 3 months, we finally went to the orthopaedist who confirmed that Gabrillian no longer had scoliosis. This was a significant progress for us because the physiotherapist could now work on his trunk and balance more.

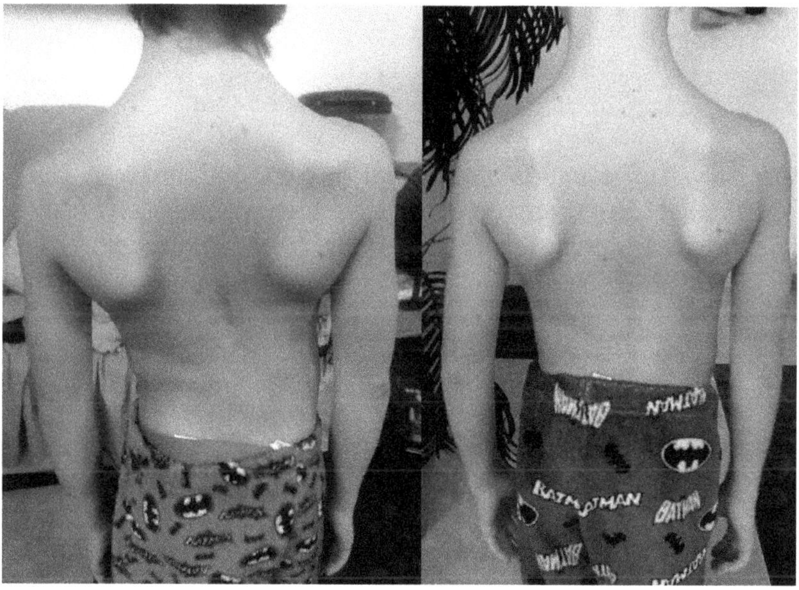

'Before and after' photos a month into therapy for postural correction.

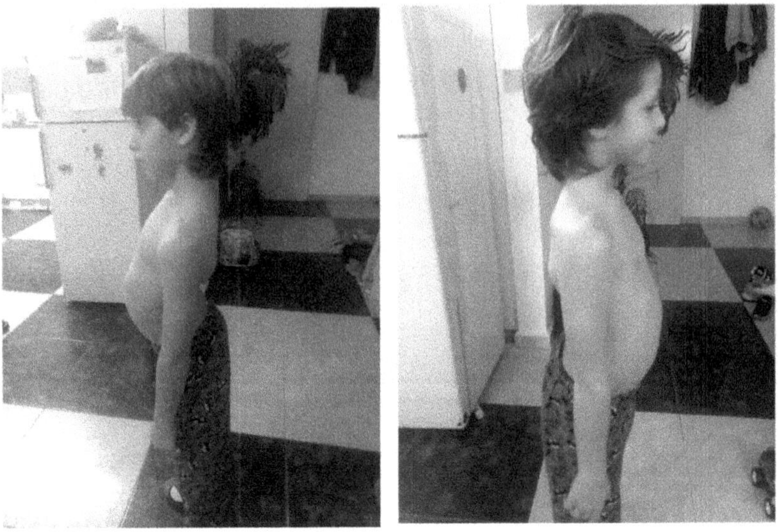

'Before and after' photos after a session of postural correction and Pons stimulation (a neurological technique), shows Gabrillian's belly is much less prominent and he is looking straight ahead."

CONCLUSION

Today, Gabrillian is a happy little boy; he can run, walk and jump. He makes friends and is accepted. He is capable of following lessons at school and really enjoys sporting activities. Our next trip to Texas will allow us to strengthen and regenerate Gabrillian's muscles using Dr Donald Rhodes' VECTTOR machine.

Our next project is to organize a detox and rehabilitation retreat in Cyprus for adults and families with children who have muscular dystrophies.

Families and individuals will benefit from all the treatments, procedures, training and assessments they need to achieve the best results."

***

Special Offer For Parents And Children

Detox Retreat in Cyprus - 10 Days to Awaken My Child's Potential'

Includes:

- 3 days of parental training
- Customised tests for your child
- Daily intensive therapies with Clémentine Ynna and a team of highly qualified specialists
- Temprana Rehabilitation
- Bio-resonance therapies
- Acupuncture therapies (optional)
- Mindset change and Visualisations
- Tai-chi

- Breathing exercises
- Accommodation and a special diet plan are provided.

For more information on the 4 or 10-day intensive programs, or for personalised coaching programs, contact us by email or via our website:

https://www.clementineynna.org or

contact@clementineynna.org

www.ingramcontent.com/pod-product-compliance
Ingram Content Group UK Ltd.
Pitfield, Milton Keynes, MK11 3LW, UK
UKHW020124290926
15471UKWH00003B/276

9 781785 55126